Calcium and the Secretory Process

Ronald P. Rubin

Department of Pharmacology
Medical College of Virginia
Richmond, Virginia

PLENUM PRESS • NEW YORK AND LONDON

Library of Congress Cataloging in Publication Data

Rubin, Ronald P
  Calcium and the secretory process.

  Bibliography: p.
  1. Calcium in the body. 2. Secretion. 3. Cyclic adenylic acid. I. Title. [DNLM: 1.
Calcium — Physiology QV276 R896c]
QP535.C2R8   612'.4   74-10557
ISBN 978-1-4757-1228-5   ISBN 978-1-4757-1226-1 (eBook)
DOI 10.1007/978-1-4757-1226-1

© 1974 Plenum Press, New York
Softcover reprint of the hardcover 1st edition 1974
A Division of Plenum Publishing Corporation
227 West 17th Street, New York, N.Y. 10011

United Kingdom edition published by Plenum Press, London
A Division of Plenum Publishing Company, Ltd.
4a Lower John Street, London, W1R 3PD, England

To

my teachers, colleagues, and students —

whose dedication to the advancement of

scientific knowledge provided the

inspiration for this project.

Preface

An enormous amount of research effort has been directed toward elucidating the mechanism by which substances are extruded from cells; and reviews have been written and symposia held in order to systematize the plethora of evidence made available. However, the approaches employed to study the secretory process have been so diverse that it is difficult, if not impossible, for one individual or even a group of individuals to keep abreast of all aspects of the field and to analyze them critically. Thus I undertook the writing of this volume with a great deal of trepidation.

In searching for some starting point, I naturally considered as my primary focus the role of calcium in the secretory process, which has occupied my research interests for the past 13 years. But since so much experimentation has been carried out on this and related topics during the last decade or two, I felt it was still necessary to visualize this venture from two alternative approaches: (1) a more general one, which would cover the subject of calcium and the secretory process from a broad perspective, but of course not in great detail, and (2) a more specific one, restricting coverage to carefully defined limits but with comprehensive analysis of limited topics. The final course undertaken appears to lie somewhere between these two extremes. Thus the scope of this volume covers a range of topics, from the general effects of calcium on a variety of biological systems to the specific role of calcium in exocytosis. The overall format incorporates a review of the pertinent literature references, with a discussion of derived conclusions. However, discussions have been limited to what is generally considered valid, and wild speculations—which in all probability will eventually be proven false—have been kept to a minimum.

The author has attempted to curtail personal bias in making as objective a presentation as possible, and it is hoped that the point of view developed is the result of careful and objective evaluation of the vast amount of scientific data that have accumulated over the years. But where bias does manifest itself, a bibliography is included so that the reader may refer to original sources or review articles to make his own judgments. However, it was not the author's purpose to have this volume become a ponderous compendium of facts, figures, and citations, which would have made it almost as difficult to read as it would have been to write. Therefore, certain references have been arbitrarily chosen to support a point to be made, although in many cases there probably are others which would be equally applicable. Some references are cited not necessarily because they are the pioneering or most definitive studies in a particular area of research, but because they provide the reader with the bibliography needed to gain an overview of a particular field. To aid the reader in this regard, review articles are cited whenever possible. Limiting the discussion is of course fraught with the danger that in the name of conciseness simplistic and even dubious conclusions may very well be drawn; and a sincere attempt has been made to avoid this pitfall.

It is the author's fervent hope that material presented in this book will be of value and interest to students of biology who wish to acquaint themselves with current trends in the field of secretory phenomena, to researchers studying various facets of the secretory process and the obviously critical but as yet incompletely defined role of calcium, and also to those who are investigating other biological processes in which calcium plays key—and possibly related—roles.

Finally, I would like to acknowledge my appreciation and extend thanks to the following individuals whose arduous endeavors helped to bring the manuscript into final form: Drs.

Robert Furchgott, Siret Jaanus, and George Weiss for reading one or more chapters and providing constructive suggestions; Mrs. Frances Woodley and Mrs. Edith Weg for typing the manuscript and correcting the all too numerous errors in grammar and punctuation; and Judi Rubin for assisting in the difficult task of preparing and systematizing the bibliography.

I also wish to express my sincere thanks to The Commonwealth Fund for its generous support in the preparation of the monograph through The Commonwealth Fund Book Program.

R.R.

Contents

CHAPTER 1

General Concepts

BIOLOGICAL IMPORTANCE OF CALCIUM

Any study of biology, even a most cursory one, is almost certain to touch on the subject of inorganic cations. Sodium and potassium are, of course, of great importance to living cells by virtue of their respective predominance in extracellular and intracellular fluids. Physiological solutions are not as rich in calcium, but the extreme biological significance of this divalent cation to plant and animal organisms has been a scientific truism for many years; for calcium is clearly implicated both in the basic organization of biological systems and in physicochemical reactions involved with many cellular functions.

A fundamental role of calcium in the constitution of biological systems relates to its presence in bone to provide the organism with required rigidity but calcium also affects cell structure and function by being indispensable for the overall integrity of tissues. The biologists of the last century were cognizant of this important fact, as exemplified by the experiments of Sidney Ringer (1890), who observed that adding calcium chloride to distilled water minimized the swelling of aquatic organisms produced by water imbibition and sustained life much longer than corresponding quantities of either sodium or potassium salts. He reasoned that calcium

1

inhibited swelling not only by influencing the direct osmotic effects of distilled water but also by somehow affecting the cement substance which binds cells together, thereby preventing the entry of water into the cells. This provided the original observation of the basic importance of calcium in many aspects of cellular adhesion, and it is now well known that in calcium-deficient media epithelial cells lose their integrity and become detached from one another; the readdition of calcium leads to a reaggregation of dissociated cells (Armstrong, 1966; Gingell *et al.*, 1970).

The permeability of a cell constitutes another very important factor in determining its behavior, and during the first half of this century physiologists and biologists also began to focus on the importance of calcium in the regulation of membrane permeability, as evidenced by its ability to interfere with cell lysis produced by osmotic or mechanical means (Lucke and McCutcheon, 1932; Davson and Danielli, 1952). It was observed that when red blood cells, for example, were placed in solutions of nonelectrolytes, such as dextrose or lactose, they rapidly lost potassium chloride and eventually hemolyzed. Sodium chloride was partially effective in delaying or preventing hemolysis, but calcium was much more effective. We now know that calcium also modulates monovalent cation permeability in excitable tissues (Brink, 1954; Frankenhaeuser and Hodgkin, 1957; Shanes, 1958), which provides the explanation for calcium control of nerve and muscle excitability, but it does not explain the mechanism for the important role of calcium in transmission of the impulse from nerve to muscle, which was demonstrated by the early experiments of Locke (1894). This classical study laid the groundwork for the subsequent investigations which eventually led to the discovery of the role of calcium in neurotransmitter release and muscle contraction.

Calcium also plays a prominent role in the chemical reactions involved with blood coagulation. Heilbrunn (1956) emphasized what he believed to be an analogous coagulative effect of calcium on the cytoplasm of primitive organisms, and he postulated that the variety of stimulant actions of calcium may be ascribed to its "coagulating" properties. In this regard, a fundamental mechanism appears to underlie cellular cytoplasmic movements in most cells (Jahn and Bovee, 1969). Examples of this phenomenon include muscle contractility in higher organisms, ameboid movement in lower forms of life, and a microtubular system in neuronal tissue which is responsible for transporting substances synthesized in cell body to the nerve terminal. Moreover, translocation of cellular organelles such as chloroplasts in plant cells and mitochondria in animal cells is brought about by cytoplasmic streaming. Protoplasmic motility seems to involve an actomyosin-like protein complex that splits high-energy phosphates; this process is also triggered by calcium ion. The ubiquitous action of calcium on protoplasmic motility will be discussed in more detail in Chapter 3 in regard to a possible explanation for its role in the secretory process.

The myriad effects of calcium on cell processes are compounded by the fact that it also regulates energy production by activating glycogenolysis (Landowne and Ritchie, 1971) and by enhancing respiration and electron transport in mitochondria (Chance, 1965), in addition to regulating the activity of innumerable enzyme systems (Rasmussen and Nagata, 1970). Thus although this monograph will emphasize the cardinal role of calcium in the mechanism whereby substances of diverse nature are extruded from cells, it is clear that its influence on the cell is widespread; and although calcium does indeed exert a direct action on the secretory process, the effects of calcium on other biological processes may indirectly influence the amount of secretory product released and can therefore scarcely be neglected.

CALCIUM DISTRIBUTION AND TISSUE CONCENTRATIONS

For the organism to carry out its varied functions—and even to survive—the calcium concentration in biological fluids must be maintained within narrow limits. The plasma calcium concentration (10 mg/100 ml)—which normally fluctuates only by ± 3%—is maintained by a number of homeostatic mechanisms, most notably parathyroid hormone, vitamin D, and thyrocalcitonin. These three substances regulate the calcium concentration as a resultant of three actions: (1) net absorption from the gut, (2) net loss through the urine, and (3) net deposition in bone. Approximately 99 % of the total body calcium is present in bone, which acts as a reservoir to maintain the requisite supply of calcium to the tissues via the circulation; even the remaining 1 % in the circulation is not all biologically active, since 50% of the plasma calcium is bound to plasma proteins.

If one endeavors to obtain information on tissue calcium concentrations, many inconsistencies are encountered. The disparities in reported values may be partially accounted for by the differences in the techniques used for the determinations. A variety of methods have been employed, including conventional spectrophotometry (Grossman and Furchgott, 1964) and fluorescence spectrophotometry (Jaanus and Rubin, 1971), as well as atomic absorption spectrophotometry (Hilmy and Somjen, 1968) and dual-wavelength spectrophotometry using the calcium complexing dye, murexide (Ohnishi and Ebashi, 1963). More recently, a photometric technique has been introduced which uses aequorin, a protein isolated from the jellyfish, which reacts with calcium to emit light (Ashley and Ridgway, 1970). Some methods, such as the fluorescence technique, determine total calcium, whereas aequorin is employed to determine ionized (free) calcium.

In evaluating data on calcium concentrations, one must consider that a portion of the ion present is not confined to parenchymal cells, but to supportive tissue as well. However, certain generalizations can still be made in regard to the calcium content of tissues. The calcium concentrations of most tissues tend to cluster around a value of $1\,\mu$mole/gram wet weight (Table I). This is true for muscle (skeletal, cardiac, and smooth) as well as peripheral nerve and brain. Glandular tissue derived from both ectoderm and neuroblasts contains similar calcium concentrations. By contrast, certain tissues which have specialized mechanisms for sequestering calcium, such as kidney and salivary glands, have higher calcium concentrations, whereas erythrocytes, which lack these mechanisms, have low concentrations (Table I). Baker and his associates (Baker, 1972) have attempted to circumvent somewhat the problem of tissue heterogeneity by measuring the calcium concentration of axoplasm after extruding it from membranous elements. They found that the axoplasm contains $400\,\mu M$ calcium;

TABLE I

Calcium Content of Various Tissues

Tissue	Calcium concentration ($\mu M/g$)	Reference
Cerebral cortex	1.2	Hilmy and Somjen (1968)
Peripheral nerve	2.9	
Muscle		
Cardiac	1.4	Grossman and Furchgott (1964)
Smooth	3.0	Goodford (1967)
Skeletal	1.5	Cosmos and Harris (1961)
Kidney		
Cortex	8.9	Cooke (1971)
Medulla	16.9	
Liver	0.3	Thiers *et al.* (1960)
Spleen	0.8	Garcia and Kirpekar (unpublished)
Salivary gland	7.3	Wallach and Schramm (1971)
Adrenal		
Cortex	1.7	Jaanus and Rubin (1971)
Medulla	2.0	
Platelets	8.0	Mürer and Holme (1970)
Erythrocytes	0.02	Harrison and Long (1968)

10 μM is diffusible but un-ionized and thought to be associated with cellular ATP, citrate, etc. Only 0.3 μM is ionized, and the remaining 300 μM is sequestered in mitochondria.

It should be emphasized that the distribution of calcium in the cell does not represent a homogeneous pool but is a complex compartmentalization, with the distribution determined by the morphological makeup of the cell (Borle, 1967; Langer, 1968). However, the compartmentalization of calcium can be arbitrarily divided up into (1) interstitial fraction; (2) membrane fractions, which include the plasma membrane systems and endoplasmic reticulum—the latter including specialized membrane systems such as the sarcoplasmic reticulum in muscle; (3) other cellular organelles, which include the mitochondria, secretory granules, and lysosomes. Calcium even binds to such ubiquitous substances as DNA and RNA, since they are highly charged anionic polyelectrolytes at neutral pH and readily form stable complexes with cations (Carr and Chang, 1971).

Most of cell calcium exists in the bound state; it is bound to the plasma membrane and the cellular membrane components, to the collagen and mucopolysaccharides of ground substance, and to many other negatively charged constituents of cells. The basis for this avid binding may, at least in part, be ascribed to the interaction between calcium and acidic phospholipids, basic constituents of membranes (Feinstein, 1964; Dawson and Hauser, 1970). Although binding to membranes accounts for some of the calcium sequestered in cells, a perhaps more important source of calcium sequestration may be the mitochondria, which provide the most important sites of bound calcium in certain systems.

REDISTRIBUTION OF CALCIUM DURING STIMULATION

While exact quantitation of each component of cell calcium is quite difficult with the techniques presently available, it is even more difficult to discern a shift in calcium from one cell compartment to another. Experiments which have employed radioactive calcium (^{45}Ca) to localize different cell fractions have shown them to be multicompartmentalized and kinetically definable into different cell fractions. Generally, there is a fraction which is readily exchangeable with extracellular medium with a half-time ($t_{\frac{1}{2}}$) of 1–5 min, a less readily exchangeable fraction with a $t_{\frac{1}{2}}$ of about 30 min, and a nonexchangeable fraction (Bianchi, 1968; Borle, 1971). A fraction may represent a summation of efflux from more than one compartment, which makes it difficult to relate these fractions to a specific cellular entity. It is even difficult to localize calcium by cell fractionation studies, due to the problem of calcium redistribution during the homogenization and centrifugation procedures.

Tracer studies may give some indication of a redistribution of calcium pools during stimulation, but even in studies involving enhanced calcium entry, caution must be used in the interpretation of data, since the magnitude of the response is not always related to the increase in calcium influx (Douglas and Poisner, 1964b; Weiss and Bianchi, 1965). However, such studies may be able to provide information as to where a critical calcium fraction is not localized. Thus if the secretory response of a given organ is diminished by the removal of calcium from the extracellular fluid, radiocalcium studies will give an approximation of the cell calcium which is not exchangeable and therefore not involved in the secretory response. However, such data may not allow one to ascertain whether the critical calcium fraction is extracellular or is in a cellular fraction which is readily exchangeable with the extracellular fluid.

In order for calcium to exert its effects, it of course must gain access to critical cellular sites, but the plasma membrane limits the entry of calcium, other cations, and permeable solutes. In most excitable cells the resting permeability to calcium is quite low, being one to three orders of magnitude less than for monovalent cations (Hodgkin and Keynes, 1957). The relatively high permeability to potassium at rest accounts for the fact that the resting membrane potential of excitable tissue and most secretory cells is determined by the ratio of the extra- and intracellular potassium concentrations (Hodgkin and Katz, 1949a). Secretory cells also appear to have enhanced resting permeability to sodium, as evidenced by the fact that the resting membrane potential of secretory cells (9–70 mV) is generally lower than that of electrically excitable cells (60–90 mV) (Table II).

Although the resting permeability of cells to calcium is considered to be low, electrical or chemical stimulation of many types of tissue is associated with a redistribution of this divalent cation. The stimulating agent may be electric current, excess potassium, or other depolarizing agents such as acetylcholine. In electrically excitable tissues, such as nerve, and cardiac and smooth muscle, stimulation is associated with an enhanced movement of calcium from the extracellular fluid across the plasma membrane into the cell. Chemical transmitter substances, especially those which penetrate cells poorly, also act to increase permeability of cell membranes to extracellular cations, including calcium. For

TABLE II

Resting Membrane Potentials of Secretory Cells

Tissue	Mean resting membrane potential (mV)	Reference
Salivary gland		
Rat parotid	−20	Schneyer et al. (1972)
Cat submaxillary	−22	Lundberg (1958)
Cat submaxillary	−21	Petersen (1972)
Pancreas		
Mouse acinar cells	−41	Dean and Matthews (1970a)
Rat acinar cells	−35	Kanno (1972)
Mouse islet cells	−20	Dean and Matthews (1970a)
Adrenal		
Rabbit, rat, kitten cortical cells	−66 to −71	Matthews (1967)
Rabbit, rat, kitten medullary cells	−20 to −32	Matthews (1967)
Gerbil medullary chromaffin cells	−29	Douglas et al. (1967a)
Thyroid		
Rat and guinea pig	−50	Woodbury and Woodbury (1963)
Rabbit	−43	Williams (1966)
Adenohypophysis		
Rat	−9	Milligan and Kraicer (1970)
Mast cells		
Rat	−14	Tasaka et al. (1970)

example, acetylcholine enhances calcium permeability in adrenal chromaffin cells (Douglas and Poisner, 1962) and in the homologous sympathetic ganglion cells (Pappano and Volle, 1966), as well as in mammalian nonmyelinated nerve fibers (Ritchie, 1965) and at the motor end-plate region (Takeuchi, 1963). Although the amount of calcium taken up during stimulation may be related to the extracellular calcium concentration, enhanced influx may not be maintained during prolonged stimulation but may decrease with time (Shanes, 1961); the inactivation of the calcium current prevents the intracellular calcium concentration from increasing to a point where it would be deleterious to the cell and may, at least in part, account for the decrease in the response commonly observed during prolonged stimulation.

The calcium currents activated following stimulation are less distinctly defined than the sodium and potassium currents. Pharmacological dissection of these currents during the nerve action potential and kinetic studies have provided evidence that the sodium and potassium channels are independent structures (Hille, 1970). Tetrodotoxin, a poison obtained from the puffer fish, specifically inhibits the more rapid and more transient increase in sodium permeability, whereas such agents as tetraethylammonium effect a selective depression of the late potassium current. During the course of the nerve action potential, calcium ion appears to pass through the membrane via two distinct sets of channels (Baker, 1972). An early transient calcium current apparently enters through the sodium gates, since it is blocked by tetrodotoxin. A later current, which does not pass through the potassium channel, manifests the properties of the calcium-dependent transmitter release mechanism, since it is insensitive to the toxin but is blocked by manganese and magnesium, which are both potent inhibitors of the release process.

It thus appears that the calcium which traverses the cell membrane to trigger the secretory process enters the cell through functionally different channels than the cations mainly responsible for carrying the current of the action potential. This conclusion is clearly substantiated by the finding in isolated adrenal chromaffin cells—which are developmental homologues of the neuron—that the local anesthetic tetracaine can specifically block the inward calcium current augmented by cholinergic agents without impeding the sodium current (Douglas and Kanno, 1967). The calcium which enters the neurons during the early phase of the action potential, though not directly involved with activation of the secretory process, could participate indirectly either by displacing cellular calcium from storage sites or by replenishing intracellular stores from which calcium can be released during stimulation. Although there is as yet no evidence for such phenomena in secretory cells, calcium redistribution during the muscle-contraction cycle may initiate such events (Chapman and Niedergerke, 1970; Ford and Podolsky, 1972).

Since calcium entry appears to be enhanced during the entire phase of the action potential, the question arises as to its contribution to the total current of the spike. Sodium is the most predominant cation, and thus is responsible for carrying most of the current, although in some excitable tissue alkaline earths such as calcium—and even large, positively charged cations—can substitute for sodium in generation of the action potential (Koketsu and Nishi, 1969). Crustacean fibers, for example, are electrically inexcitable or give feeble graded responses when kept in solutions of normal saline, but elicit all-or-none action potentials by replacing external sodium by calcium, strontium, or onium ions (Fatt and Ginsborg, 1958). Calcium also appears to be responsible for carrying some of the current in adrenal chromaffin cells (Douglas *et al.*, 1967b) and in the β cells of pancreatic islets (Dean and Matthews, 1970b), as well as in certain smooth (Bulbring and Tomita, 1970) and cardiac muscle preparations (Niedergerke and Orkand, 1966; Reuter, 1970). However, the large increases in calcium influx attending stimulation of secretory cells may not provide enough current to be considered an important component of the electrical changes which accompany the response. But whether or not calcium contributes to electrical events in secretory systems may be only of heuristic interest, since gross electrical changes across the cell membrane are not required for the initiation of the secretory process as long as specific effects on calcium distribution are brought about by stimulation. The idea that electrical activity can be uncoupled from secretion will be documented by evidence obtained from different tissues, demonstrating that chemical or electrical activation of the secretory process can occur in the absence of any discernible sodium current, or when the cell is completely depolarized by excess potassium, *as long as calcium is present in the bathing medium.*

Although a transmembrane flux of extracellular calcium may be the triggering event in many systems, there are data from other systems to indicate that the origin of calcium released during stimulation may be the result of a translocation of cellular calcium.

The prototype tissue where such an event occurs is skeletal muscle, where electrical impulses and chemical agents, such as caffeine, exert their primary action on intracellular membrane systems to displace a bound form of calcium (Nayler, 1966; Bianchi, 1968). Since most of the cellular calcium exists in the bound state, it seems reasonable to contemplate that at least certain substances initiate secretion by acting on calcium-storing structures to release bound calcium. And indeed there is evidence to indicate that stimulation of the secretory process in some glands may be effected by altering the state of bound cellular calcium. This appears to be the situation in regard to the action of pituitary trophic hormones on the adrenal cortex (Jaanus and Rubin, 1971) and thyroid gland (Williams, 1972b), as well as in the submaxillary and parotid salivary glands (Nielsen and Petersen, 1972; Batzri and Selinger, 1973).

The locus of calcium released during activation may depend on the type of stimulation as well as the tissue involved. The notion that different stimulating agents acting on the same system initiate activation by affecting different calcium fractions gains favor by the consistently reported finding of a differential sensitivity of certain systems to calcium deprivation on exposure to a variety of stimulating agents. For example, in the adrenal medulla, after the onset of calcium-free perfusion the secretory response to excess potassium is lost long before the response to acetylcholine or to sympathomimetic amines (Rubin, 1970). A similar phenomenon has been reported in various muscle preparations. After the introduction of a calcium-free medium, contractile responses to excess potassium are lost more rapidly than responses to acetylcholine (Edman and Schild, 1962). Moreover, in skeletal muscle the responses to excess potassium in the calcium-free deprived media can be temporarily maintained by certain divalent cations, such as nickel and cobalt (Frank, 1962). These cations are thought to act by displacing a calcium fraction bound to the sarcoplasmic reticulum. However, whether the critical calcium fraction is extracellular or cellular, translocation of this cation is a fundamental requirement for many physiological processes, including secretion and contraction.

Although the primary action of many stimulating agents results in a mobilization of free or bound calcium the reader should not infer that this is always the case. Electrical and chemical stimulation do bring about changes in membrane permeability to one or more ionic species, and, depending on the selective change in permeability, the net result may be depolarization or hyperpolarization, depending on the cation(s) or anion(s) involved. For example, if there is a specific increase in permeability to potassium and/or chloride ion, as has been observed in salivary glands after stimulation, the result will be hyperpolarization (Scheyner *et al.*, 1972). Under these conditions, it seems highly unlikely that there would be an increased inward calcium current, but calcium might still be involved in the membrane effects which lead to the specific changes in membrane permeability. The explanation for the changes occurring at the receptor level which result in characteristic ionic events may be related to the specific composition of the membrane phospholipids which cause them to respond in their distinct way after stimulation.

REGULATION OF CELL CALCIUM

In light of the obvious importance of calcium movements during cell activity, the calcium concentration at specific cellular sites might increase indefinitely with every stimulation unless there were some mechanism for its removal or sequestration. The continuous presence of excess calcium in the intracellular environment may lead to excessive or prolonged activity, or to deleterious effects such as depression of neuronal excitability (Watanabe and Tasaki, 1971), permeability increase to intracellular potassium (Kregenow and Hoffman, 1972; Meech, 1972), or depression of active transport mechanisms through inhibition of Na-K-ATPase (Dunham and Glynn, 1961), the enzyme responsible for maintaining the sodium–potassium gradient across the plasma membrane. It has already been mentioned that the free cellular calcium concentration is very low (10^{-5} to 10^{-7} M). However, if the calcium concentration were determined solely by the Donnan ratio, the concentration should be somewhere between 0.1 and 10 mM. It is therefore obvious that the distribution of calcium in intracellular compartments is not determined by simple passive distribution.

Binding

One means whereby the biological activity of calcium is curtailed is by sequestration, and there is a plethora of evidence from both biological and artificial membrane systems indicating that calcium avidly binds to membrane fractions (Carvalho, 1966; Dawson and Hauser, 1970). These membrane fractions may be the plasma membrane (Mazia, 1940; Forstner and Manery, 1971; Madeira and Carvalho, 1972) or cellular membrane systems (endoplasmic reticulum) (Meisde *et al.*, 1970). The binding of calcium to the microsomal fraction of nervous tissue (Yoshida *et al.*, 1966; Robinson and Lust, 1968) resembles calcium accumulation by sarcoplasmic reticulum of skeletal and cardiac muscle (Weber *et al.*, 1967; Ebashi and Endo, 1968), and certainly accounts for some of calcium binding which takes place during activity; however, the exact source of the microsomal fraction obtained by high-speed centrifugation has not been clearly established and may represent components of the plasma membrane as well as cellular membrane fractions (Bondani and Karler, 1970). A portion of calcium accumulation by membrane components depends on metabolism (active transport), but some accumulation occurs more rapidly and does not depend on metabolic activity, i.e., simple binding (Yoshida *et al.*, 1966; Palmer and Posey, 1970).

Calcium uptake is also a general property of mitochondria, where there is a stoichiometric coupling of calcium accumulation to electron transport (Chance, 1965; Lehninger, 1970). The avidity with which calcium is transported into mitochondria is exemplified by studies showing that a major portion of radiocalcium injected *in vivo* finds its way into the mitochondrial fraction of tissues (Patriarca and Carafoli, 1968); moreover, calcium is taken up in preference to ADP (Lehninger, 1970). Thus calcium uptake appears to have primacy over phosphorylation of ADP, which has been generally thought to be the primary function of mitochondria. The importance of mitochondria in calcium binding, however, varies from tissue to tissue (Carafoli and Lehninger, 1971). In squid giant axon it appears to be responsible for binding most of the cell calcium (Baker, 1972). Although the mitochondrial and microsomal fractions of adrenal medulla (see Poisner,

1973) and salivary gland (Selinger *et al.*, 1970) also avidly bind calcium, the secretory granules of these glands manifest very high calcium concentrations (Borowitz *et al.*, 1965; Wallach and Schramm, 1971), indicating that these organelles also play a prime role in maintaining the free calcium level of their respective cells at very low levels.

Exchange Diffusion

Not only is cellular calcium inactivated by binding to intracellular structures, but it is also removed from cells by exchanging with extracellular cations. Stimulation of certain secretory organs, such as the neurohypophysis and adrenal medulla, which have been labeled with radiocalcium shows a marked enhancement of calcium efflux (Douglas and Poisner, 1964b; Rubin *et al.*, 1967) (Fig. 1a). This increase in calcium efflux—which depends on the presence of calcium in the external medium—is most prominent in tissues where extracellular calcium is utilized in the secretory process and where stimulation is associated with a large increase in calcium influx. Not all calcium-dependent secretory systems manifest this increase in calcium efflux following stimulation. In the adrenal cortex, which utilizes cellular calcium for its secretory activity, stimulation in a calcium-containing or calcium-deprived medium is associated with a decrease in calcium efflux (Jaanus and Rubin, 1971), which indicates a translocation of cell calcium from a more readily exchangeable fraction to one that is less readily exchangeable, rather than a transmembrane calcium flux (Fig. 1b).

Calcium–calcium exchange takes place even in the resting state, for radiocalcium is lost from tissues more rapidly when there is "cold" calcium in the extracellular medium than when there is not (Shanes and Bianchi, 1959). The calcium–calcium exchange obviously does little to bring about a lowering of intracellular calcium, but it does succeed in preventing the calcium levels in cells from rising to toxic concentrations and helps to keep calcium metabolism in a dynamic state.

Baker and his colleagues have also provided evidence for a linking of calcium efflux coupled to sodium influx, i.e., an exchange of intracellular calcium for extracellular sodium (Baker, 1972).

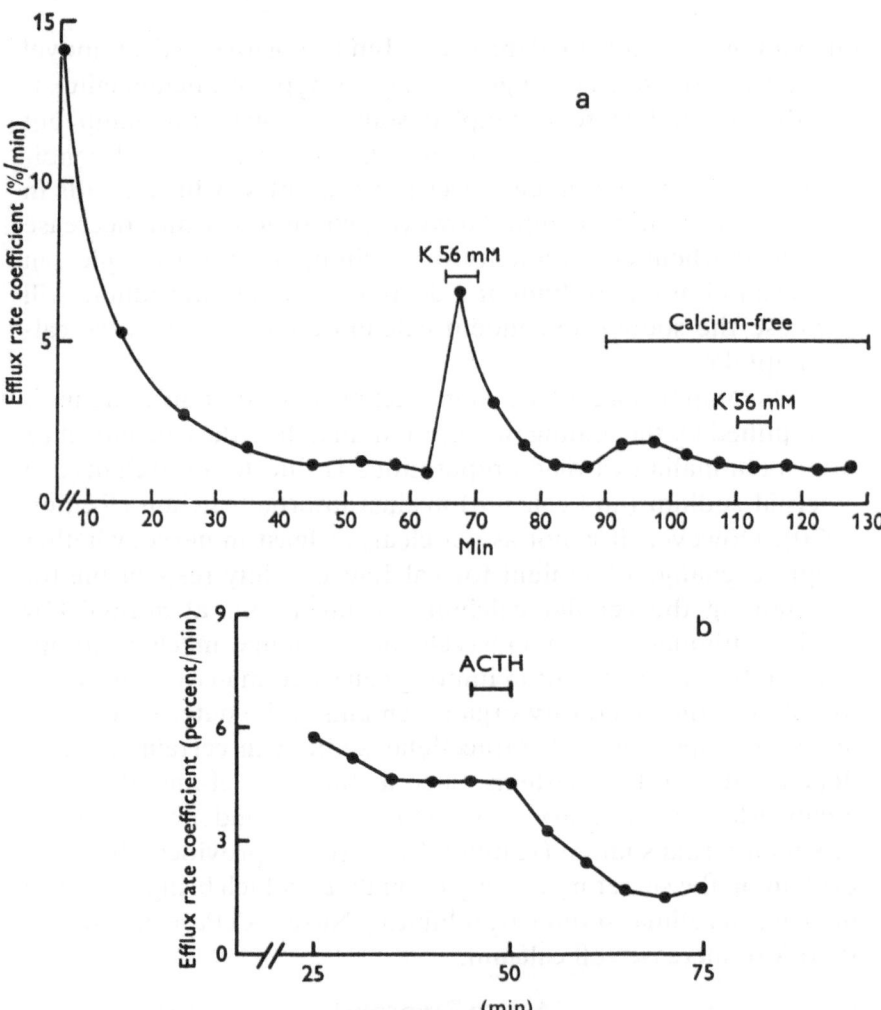

Fig. 1(a) Stimulant effect of excess potassium on ^{45}Ca efflux from isolated rat neurohypophyses and its dependence on calcium (Douglas and Poisner, 1964b). (b) The effect of ACTH on ^{45}Ca efflux from the cat adrenal gland perfused *in situ* with calcium-free Locke's solution (Jaanus and Rubin, 1971).

This type of exchange, which has been demonstrated in squid and crab nerve (Baker, 1972), in smooth and cardiac muscle preparations (Goodford, 1967; Reuter and Seitz, 1968), and in brain (Bull and Trevor, 1972; Stahl and Swanson, 1972), is not sensitive to ouabain or to potassium deprivation but is sensitive to the removal of external sodium. This suggests that this type of calcium efflux is not directly linked to a coupled sodium–potassium pump but involves sodium–calcium exchange. Under physiological conditions, nerve stimulation enhances sodium entry, which results in loss of intracellular calcium. However, conditions which decrease the electrochemical gradient for sodium, as, for example, an increase in internal sodium or a decrease in external sodium, will decrease the sodium-dependent calcium efflux and increase calcium uptake.

The importance of calcium exchange in certain systems is exemplified by the finding that more than half of the calcium efflux from mammalian cardiac preparations is due to an exchange of external sodium (and calcium) against internal calcium (Reuter, 1970). However, it is not as yet clear, at least in nerve, whether simple exchange of sodium for calcium is solely responsible for maintaining the cellular calcium concentrations at normal low levels. Although the sodium–calcium exchange mechanism appears to be a prime factor in limiting cell calcium in excitable cells, its role in other secretory organs remains to be determined. The apparent importance of intracellular sodium in certain calcium-dependent secretory systems, such as the adrenal medulla, pancreatic islets, and salivary gland, points to a dependence of calcium flux on internal sodium (Rubin, 1970). It also provides a basis for explaining the secretory activity of ouabain, which brings about an increase in cellular sodium by inhibiting Na-K-ATPase, and would therefore increase cell calcium.

Active Transport

The erythrocyte maintains a very low level of intracellular calcium by an active transport mechanism which does not involve binding to membranes or cell organelles or exchange diffusion. A calcium-activated ATPase system has been demonstrated that is distinct from the sodium–calcium exchange diffusion process demonstrable in excitable tissue and from the ATPase system responsible for sodium transport but that is similar to the calcium uptake system in the endoplasmic reticulum, which also involves a calcium-activated ATPase and ATP hydrolysis (Schatzmann,

1970). The dependence of the sodium–calcium exchange process on energy results indirectly from the energy requirement of sodium transport, which maintains the necessary concentration of sodium between the extracellular medium and the cell. On the other hand, calcium extrusion by the red blood cell requires ATP directly and is independent of the occurrence of sodium transport. Thus, by means of ion exchange diffusion or by active transport, cells can bring about an energy-dependent net extrusion of calcium.

This raises the question as to whether secretory cells maintain low levels of cell calcium by an energy-dependent process. Calcium-activated ATPases have been demonstrated in a number of secretory organs, and their physiological function(s) has not been defined (Rubin, 1970). Moreover, whereas calcium entry into cells is presumed to be passive down an electrochemical gradient, calcium efflux is generally considered to be an active process, as evidenced by the inhibition of calcium efflux from brain by metabolic inhibitors (Cooke and Robinson, 1971). On the other hand, metabolic inhibitors may cause an increase in calcium efflux by releasing calcium from such binding sites as the mitochondria (Blaustein and Hodgkin, 1969; Carafoli *et al.*, 1969); so the use of metabolic inhibitors to help elucidate the mechanism of calcium efflux from cells will not allow clear-cut conclusions to be drawn.

CALCIUM AND MEMBRANE PERMEABILITY

Up to now, emphasis has focused on the idea that the cell activity in response to stimulation is associated with a redistribution of extra- and intracellular calcium. In secretory cells this translocation is associated with an enhanced release of secretory product. Since the specialized function of a secretory organ is in many ways a reflection of the general factors affecting the activity of its cells, as, for example, their permeability properties, such general factors must also be considered.

Compelling evidence to support the concept that calcium plays a crucial role in modulating cell permeability is not only the irrefutable association of calcium with cell membrane fractions but also the variety of evidence from many different biological systems and artificial membrane models, which clearly demonstrates that calcium controls the permeability of membranes to cations, water, and macromolecules (Lucke and McCutcheon, 1932; Davson and Danielli, 1952; Shanes, 1958; Manery, 1966). The early biologists, working on more primitive biological systems, noted the importance of calcium (and other divalent cations) in maintaining the normal permeability of cells by protecting against lysis by osmotic, mechanical, and pH effects (Lucke and McCutcheon, 1932). Exposure of brain or liver slices to calcium-free media increases cell permeability, as evidenced by the loss of cell potassium, protein, ADP, and cytoplasmic enzymes such as lactic dehydrogenase and aldolase (Manery, 1966).

The action of calcium on cell membranes may be viewed as a stabilizing action. The term "membrane stabilization" was originated by Guttman in 1940, when she found that calcium reduced the depolarizing effect of excess potassium on the nerve membrane. As the calcium concentration is increased, the nerve becomes less responsive to stimulating agents, although the resting potential undergoes little change. Other divalent cations, such as magnesium and strontium, produce the same phenomenon. Shanes (1958) later presented a more extended classification of stabilizing agents to include any agent which inhibited any change in the resting membrane potential. Local anesthetics also fall into the classification of stabilizing agents, and they, like calcium, avidly bind to natural and artificial membrane systems and interact with acidic phospholipids in a stoichiometric manner (Feinstein, 1964; Papahadjopoulos, 1972). Moreover, they can protect against the increase in permeability attending the removal of calcium from the medium (Blaustein and Goldman, 1966). Feinstein (1964) suggested that local anesthetics can replace calcium at membrane anionic sites and thereby inhibit ion flux; however, although local anesthetics can stabilize the membrane like calcium, they—unlike calcium—inhibit the generation of the action potential.

If the barrier properties of the cell membrane are maintained by calcium, then calcium deprivation might be expected to alter normal ionic gradients, resulting in a change in the electrical properties of excitable tissue. Indeed, the early neurophysiologists noted that calcium deprivation resulted in an increase in the excitability of nerve and muscle (cf. Brink, 1954). The threshold for inducing electrical activity is markedly reduced and spontaneous firing is observed in the absence of calcium, although release of neurotransmitter is depressed. A decrease in the resting membrane potential is demonstrable in many excitable tissues after calcium deprivation (Shanes, 1958), and Frankenhauser and Hodgkin (1957) have estimated that in the squid axon a fivefold decrease in calcium concentration is similar to depolarization of 10–15 mV. One may thus generalize that calcium excess and lack may be likened to anodal and cathodal stimulation, respectively.

The introduction of the voltage clamp technique in the 1950s enabled further elucidation of calcium action on the excitable membrane. Frankenhaeuser and Hodgkin (1957) demonstrated that changes in the calcium concentration in the external medium affect both the early, more transient inward sodium current and the later, longer-lasting outward potassium current. They showed that in the presence of low calcium a smaller depolarization step is required to reach a given conductance change; conversely, an increase in the calcium concentration results in a larger depolarization being necessary to reach a given conductance change.

Not only can calcium regulate the size and shape of the action potential by affecting the size and extent of the inward sodium current, but it is also responsible for carrying some of the inward current, at least in certain excitable tissues (Koketsu and Nishi, 1969; Bulbring and Tomita, 1970; Reuter, 1970). Thus when evaluating the role of calcium in the release of neurotransmitter substances, one must always consider its indirect actions as the result of its membrane effects on cell permeability and tissue excitability. The distinction between the effects of calcium on tissue excitability and on the secretory process is made clear by the actions of certain other divalent cations, such as magnesium and manganese, which, in the absence of calcium, will maintain normal tissue excitability by manifesting calcium-like effects on tissue permeability (Maizels, 1956; Frankenhaeuser and Meves, 1958; Rojas *et al.*, 1969) but will not support secretion (Rubin, 1970; Meiri and Rahamimoff, 1972).

The role of calcium in regulating membrane permeability is probably related to its characteristic property to interact with anionic sites on the membrane (Shanes, 1958; Tobias, 1964)—more specifically with acidic phospholipids (Abramson *et al.*, 1964; Feinstein, 1964) and ATP (Abood, 1966), which are important constituents of cell membranes. Phospholipid–calcium interactions appear most critical for normal membrane integrity (Cuthbert, 1967), although ATP may also be very important, since it can substitute for calcium in maintaining normal permeability characteristics of neurons (Kuperman *et al.*, 1967); moreover, the chelation stability of the calcium–ATP complex is quite high, being of the same order as the calcium–citrate complex (Hodgkin and Keynes, 1957; Rubin, 1963). A membrane may be regarded as a site for cation exchange where the charge density and cation size may be important factors in determining the affinity of a cation for a given site. Calcium ions, having a much greater affinity for the negatively charged membrane sites than monovalent cations (Carvalho, 1966; Dawson and Hauser, 1970), play the primary role in regulating the relative impermeability of cells to ions and larger molecules at rest.

Since calcium plays a crucial role in regulating the relative impermeability of cells in the resting state, it therefore follows that the permeability changes which follow membrane stimulation also involve calcium. The concept has been advanced many times that the key process during cell stimulation or activation is a displacement of calcium from certain negatively charged membrane sites, which causes macromolecules to undergo a conformational change leading to an increase in permeability (Tobias, 1964; Douglas, 1965; Somlyo and Somlyo, 1968). Although direct evidence for this molecular event is still lacking, all of the indirect evidence summarized herein points to this conclusion, as well as the finding that calcium binding to the receptor area is an important factor in receptor reactivity to chemical stimulation (Paton and Rothschild, 1965; Tuttle and Moran, 1969; Manthey, 1972).

ION ANTAGONISMS

When evaluating the role of calcium in secretion and other types of cellular activity, its relation to other cations must always be considered. The ability of sodium and potassium to antagonize many of the effects of calcium in a variety of plant and animal cells has been known since the last century (cf. Hober, 1945). In 1883 Sidney Ringer noted that sodium and potassium oppose the stimulant effect of calcium on the heart. More recent work has shown that the mechanism of this antagonism is the depression of the rate of calcium entry into the heart (Lüttgau and Niedergerke, 1958). In nerve, when external sodium is reduced, calcium influx increases and calcium efflux decreases—the axon gaining calcium (Baker, 1972). This increase in calcium entry during sodium deprivation is produced by the same mechanism responsible for calcium extrusion via sodium–calcium exchange. In certain secretory systems, and under certain conditions, sodium and potassium deprivation enhance the stimulant effects of calcium (cf. Rubin, 1970), although an increase in calcium uptake has so far not been directly demonstrated under these conditions.

In order to explain the competition of divalent and monovalent cations for entry into cells, one would have to have a clear picture as to how inorganic ions penetrate cell membranes. Do ions enter the cell through pores in the membrane, or are there carriers which transport the ions? Depending on which mechanism exists, cations will compete for entry through pore sites or transport sites. An elucidation of the permeability properties of biological membranes in terms of a pore acting as the pathway for the lipid-soluble cation has been presented from the work of Solomon (1962) on red-blood cells, and by Koefoed-Johnsen and Ussing (1953) on the hormone-sensitive toad bladder. The permeability changes associated with activation of the inhibitory postsynaptic potential in cat spinal motoneurons are also in keeping with the pore structure hypothesis (Coombs et al., 1955). Permeable anions, when injected intracellularly, change hyperpolarization to depolarization, since the electrochemical gradient is altered so that the negatively charged ions flow from inside to outside. Moreover, the ability of the anions to penetrate the activated inhibitory postsynaptic membrane is related to their relative hydrated sizes, which is in harmony with the idea of a pore or sieve structure.

Despite evidence that cell membranes have pores or channels through which ions enter and leave, other available data make it difficult to explain ion antagonisms simply in terms of competition for entry. The pharmacological dissection of ionic currents with the use of such agents as tetrodotoxin and tetraethylammonium supports the existence of independent channels for the flow of potassium and sodium ions (Hille, 1970). Calcium currents are demonstrable during the entire sequence of conductance changes of sodium and potassium, but the apparent critical calcium current for triggering the secretory process does not enter the neuron through either the sodium or the potassium channels (Baker, 1972). In adrenal chromaffin cells, which have the same embryological ancestry as neuronal tissue, the inward calcium current required for catecholamine release also enters through channels functionally distinct from the inward sodium current (Douglas and Kanno, 1967). Moreover, lowering the sodium concentration of the medium bathing isolated neurohypophyses augments secretion but does not enhance calcium entry (Douglas and Poisner, 1964b). One must therefore consider the possibility that ionic events are interrelated in other ways.

Competition of membrane fractions for calcium and monovalent cations indicates that they function as cation exchangers, with the cations competing for the same binding sites (Wilbrandt and Koller, 1948; Koketsu *et al.*, 1964; Diamond and Goldberg, 1971). In tissues where calcium bound to membranous elements is critical for stimulation, a decrease in cell sodium or potassium may cause an increase in the amount of calcium bound to the membrane fractions and result in an increase in the amount of calcium released during stimulation. Alternatively, a decrease in calcium rebinding after release could theoretically lead to an increase in calcium-mediated stimulation. Calcium uptake into mitochondria depends on the relative concentrations of sodium and potassium (Dransfeld *et al.*, 1969), and a decrease in the cell concentration of one or both of these cations may lead to an increase in the free cellular calcium concentration due to a decrease in the calcium-sequestering activity of mitochondria. The resulting increase in free cellular calcium could lead to enhanced activity.

Cell calcium levels are determined not only by enhancement of calcium entry but also by the rate at which it is extruded from cells. Thus cell calcium may be augmented not only by an increase in influx but also by a slowing of efflux. Calcium efflux will depend on the amount of calcium and other cations in the cell and partly on the counter-ions outside the cell which are transported inward by the coupling mechanism as calcium is transported outward. For example, a lowering of the external potassium leads to a rise in the internal sodium concentration in nerve and red blood cells by inhibiting the sodium pump. In nerve, an increase in internal sodium leads to a decrease in calcium efflux, and possibly to an increase in calcium influx (Baker, 1972). Thus changes in the distribution of monovalent cation can lead not only to an increase in calcium uptake but also to a slowing of calcium efflux, and either of these phenomena can lead to a net increase in cell calcium. These possibilities are presented not to complicate the view of ion antagonisms but merely to point out that ion interactions occur at a variety of levels and must therefore be viewed from a number of perspectives.

SUMMARY AND CONCLUSIONS

In this chapter, an attempt has been made to lay the foundation for describing the actions of calcium on specific secretory systems by reviewing the mechanisms for controlling its distribution in biological systems. The compartmentalization of calcium is complex, with calcium being unequally distributed through various extra- and intracellular compartments. The free calcium concentration is very low, which is at least partially explained by its avid binding to membrane systems. Electrical or chemical stimulation probably involves the dissociation of a phospholipid–calcium complex which results in a transient increase in intracellular calcium and is responsible for producing the cellular response. Even when chemical or electrical stimulation is associated with an increase in calcium entry, a proportionate increase in calcium efflux may occur, which would preclude the demonstration of a net change in cell calcium. This is more than fortuitous, since a sustained increase in cell calcium may lead to continuous activity such as maintained high rates of secretion or deleterious effects such as loss of tissue excitability. Also, the ability of calcium to bind avidly to membranous components of cells under normal conditions limits the increase in free calcium in the cell and allows a more rapid termination of calcium action. Thus the intracellular calcium concentration is controlled by sequestration of free intracellular calcium by binding to the endoplasmic reticulum, mitochondria, and other cell organelles, and by extrusion of calcium to the extracellular fluid by cation exchange or active transport.

The secretory process—with which we will be primarily concerned—may be viewed as consisting of two major events: membrane excitation and the molecular events directly associated with the release process. In subsequent chapters emphasis will focus on the mechanism whereby calcium couples the membrane events which lead to the secretory response. However, when considering the varied actions of calcium, it must be kept in mind that nature has endowed this cation with the ability not only to couple membrane excitation with the response but also to help modulate its own activity by controlling the degree of responsiveness to stimulating agents as the result of its membrane-stabilizing action.

CHAPTER 2

Action of Calcium on the Secretory Process

CHOLINERGIC NEURONS, CHROMAFFIN CELLS, AND NEUROSECRETORY CELLS

Historical Background

The chronology of events dictates that a discussion of the role of calcium in secretory mechanisms should begin with the cholinergic nervous system, for there is no doubt that this was the system where definitive studies implicating calcium as a regulator of neurotransmitter release were first conducted. In actuality, evidence for the involvement of calcium in acetylcholine release was presented many years before acetylcholine was identified as the chemical transmitter at cholinergic junctions. It was in 1894 that Locke immersed the frog sartorius muscle, with its attached nerve, in a saline solution lacking calcium. After 15–20 min the muscle failed to respond when its nerve was stimulated, although it did contract to direct stimulation. The addition of a small amount of calcium to the bath restored the response to nerve stimulation. The significance of this classical experiment, which established the importance of calcium in transmission of excitation from nerve to muscle, had to await the discovery by Loewi (1921, 1945) that the

25

vagus nerve liberates a chemical substance which he termed "Vagus-stoff" before acetylcholine was identified as the chemical transmitter at the neuromuscular junction and autonomic ganglia. It was with these two cholinergic systems—as a consequence of the studies of Harvey and MacIntosh and of Bernard Katz and his associates—that the role of calcium in the release of acetylcholine was first clearly established.

In 1940 Harvey and MacIntosh, using the eserinized isolated cat cervical sympathetic ganglion, showed that when calcium was removed from the perfusion medium the release of acetylcholine from the preganglionic nerve endings either during nerve stimulation or after the injection of potassium was either greatly diminished or completely abolished (Fig. 2). These investigators ascribed the effects of calcium deprivation to a direct effect on the release reaction and not to an effect on impulse conduction, since they noted that calcium lack produced hyperexcitability of the neuronal elements although synaptic transmission was blocked. Katz and his associates (cf. Katz, 1958, 1969) have very productively employed the frog neuromuscular junction for studying transmitter release, despite the fact that acetylcholine is not measured directly. Using microelectrode techniques, they have demonstrated that the miniature end-plate potentials represent basic units (quanta) of transmitter activity and that the end-plate potential consists of a summation of such quanta. In quantifying transmitter release, either by determining the mean number of quanta released per nerve impulse (quantal content) or measuring the amplitude of the end-plate potential, it was established by comprehensive and careful investigation that calcium plays an essential and direct role in the release reaction at the amphibian neuromuscular junction. The effects of calcium were ascribed to its ability to increase the probability of release of quanta of acetylcholine during depolarization by nerve impulses.

While recognizing the pioneering efforts of the investigators on cholinergic systems—and the importance of their findings cannot be overstated—the endeavors of another investigator, William Douglas, should be given as much—or even more —recognition, for it was he who, realizing an underlying similarity in the basic machinery of the cell, had the perspicacity to transform

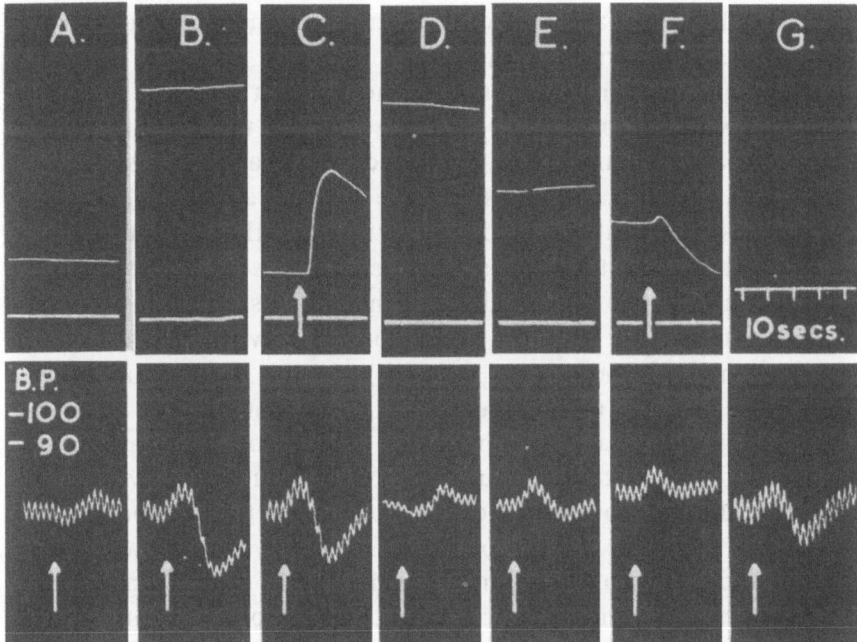

Fig. 2. Effect of calcium deprivation on acetylcholine release from the perfused superior cervical ganglion of the cat. The upper traces show nictitating membrane contractions, and the lower traces show the amount of acetylcholine released during the corresponding periods by the depressor effect of the venous effluent on cat blood pressure. (A) No stimulation, (B) maximal preganglionic nerve stimulation, (C) injection of KCl, (D–F) perfusion with calcium-free Locke's solution, (D) no stimulation, (E) maximal preganglionic stimulation 10 min later, (F) injection of KCl, (G) effect of injection of acetylcholine on cat blood pressure (Harvey and MacIntosh, 1940).

the concept of the role of calcium from that of a mere factor in acetylcholine release to one of a general mediator of secretory mechanisms (cf. Douglas, 1968). Not only did he extrapolate the findings obtained from cholinergic nerves to the secretory cells of the adrenal medulla, but he also extended his observations to the neurosecretory cells of the neurohypophysis, and finally to the submaxillary salivary gland. Moreover, his initial studies were responsible for spurring other workers to investigate the role of calcium on a variety of secretory systems, so that during the last 10 years substantial evidence has accumulated to provide convincing proof of the very basic role of calcium in the mechanism whereby substances are extruded from cells.

Scientific progress depends on the prudent selection of a basic problem which is susceptible to being solved at the current stage of scientific advancement and the selection of a proper system to study this problem. Douglas saw the role of calcium in secretory systems as a general one, and initially selected the adrenal medulla as the system to test his thesis. The medulla was for several reasons an excellent choice for carrying out this initial study. Embryologically related to the neuron, where previous work on the role of calcium had already been carried out, this endocrine organ, however, has the advantage that it does not exhibit electrical excitability, so that the important effects of calcium on the properties of excitable tissue previously alluded to would not obscure the interpretation of the action of this cation on the secretory process. Moreover, it was well known from the studies of Blaschko and Welch (1953) and Hillarp et al. (1953) that the medulla contains large stores of preformed catecholamine sequestered within specific cellular organelles which have a slow rate of turnover. Thus any effects of calcium observed could be presumed to be solely on the release process per se and not an indirect effect via hormone synthesis; it will be seen that this is a major problem in other secretory systems, as, for example, the adrenal cortex.

The evidence which had accumulated up to about 1960 indicated that in the adrenal medulla acetylcholine puts into motion a train of unknown events leading to the release of catecholamines. Yet even at that time it was known from the work of Katz and his associates (cf. Katz, 1958) that at the motor end plate acetylcholine acted on the outer surface of the plasma membrane to enhance membrane permeability to common species of extracellular cation. The investigations on cholinergic nerves had already established the importance of calcium for transmitter release, so Douglas reasoned that acetylcholine brought about catecholamine release from the adrenal by causing an enhancement of calcium uptake into the chromaffin cell.

With the aid of the author (who was a graduate student at the time) and Siret Jaanus—who quickly mastered and perfected the technique of adrenal perfusion—William Douglas set out to prove his theory (Douglas and Rubin, 1961, 1963). It was an exciting October day in 1960 in the Pharmacology Laboratory at the Albert Einstein College of Medicine when a cat adrenal gland was perfused, first with calcium-containing Locke's solution and then with calcium-free Locke's solution, and each time the gland was stimulated with acetylcholine. The effluent was collected, and the catecholamine assay was ready to be carried out.

Remember, now, this was 1960, and chemical methods for determining catecholamines were still being developed. Besides, much of Douglas's training had taken place in England, where, under the guidance of such stalwarts as Sir Henry Dale, Gaddum, and Feldberg, bioassay techniques had been developed for identifying and quantitating biological substances. So the rabbit aortic strip—the preparation of which, up to that time, Robert Furchgott (1960) had utilized so successfully for studying drug–receptor mechanisms—was employed to carry out the assay of the adrenal perfusate.

This smooth muscle preparation is sensitive to minute quantities of catecholamine, so it was not surprising when the segments of rabbit aorta suspended in the water bath responded to an injection of the acetylcholine-containing perfusate with a contraction which deflected the pen of the recorder off scale. Now the critical moment had arrived, and the three of us exulted when the piece of aorta failed to contract after a similar volume of acetylcholine-containing, calcium-free perfusate was added to the bath. This part of the experiment had answered the question as to whether or not calcium was required for catecholamine release induced by acetylcholine (Fig. 3).

When the experiment was continued to ascertain whether the effect of calcium deprivation was reversible, another interesting and very significant phenomenon was observed. The readdition of calcium to the perfusion medium—that is, switching from calcium-free to calcium-containing Locke's solution in the absence of acetylcholine or any other stimulating agent—produced a huge outpouring of medullary catecholamine (Fig. 4). This finding indicated that not only was calcium required for catecholamine release, but also its action was able to initiate secretion.

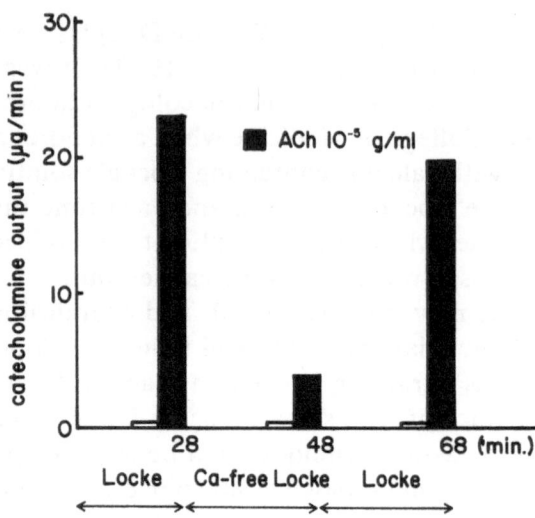

Fig. 3. The inhibitory effect of calcium deprivation on catecholamine release from the perfused cat adrenal gland in response to acetylcholine (ACh) (Douglas and Rubin 1961).

   The mechanism of the direct stimulatory effect of calcium requires some explanation, because it helps to understand certain basic physiological principles. Remembering that calcium is of great importance in controlling membrane permeability, it was reasoned that during calcium deprivation the permeability of the chromaffin cell is increased, and when calcium is returned to the perfusion medium it is able to enter the interior of the chromaffin cell to trigger the secretory process. One might therefore ask, does not magnesium have stabilizing properties similar to calcium, and would not its presence in the Locke's solution prevent any increase in permeability in the absence of calcium? This is a valid question and would have presented difficulties in interpreting the direct stimulating effect of calcium if magnesium had been present in the Locke's solution; however, fortuitously, the Locke's solution initially employed did not contain magnesium, so the stimulant effect of calcium was demonstrable. Indeed, when magnesium was added to the calcium-free solution, secretion was not enhanced, and the ability of calcium to directly trigger the secretory mechanism was abolished (Fig. 4).

The specificity of the calcium requirement was further established by subsequent experiments which showed that sodium and potassium are not required in the release process but perfusion with either sodium- or potassium-free Locke's solution actually enhances acetylcholine-induced catecholamine secretion. Not only is calcium required for secretion, but it is also a sufficient condition for release, since isotonic sucrose plus 2 mM calcium chloride provides an adequate perfusion medium for demonstrating the secretory response to acetylcholine. Additional studies showed that the secretory response to acetylcholine is related to the calcium concentration of the perfusion medium (up to 17.6 mM) and is associated with an increase in the rate of calcium uptake into the medulla. Moreover, magnesium, a well-known calcium antagonist in other biological systems, competitively

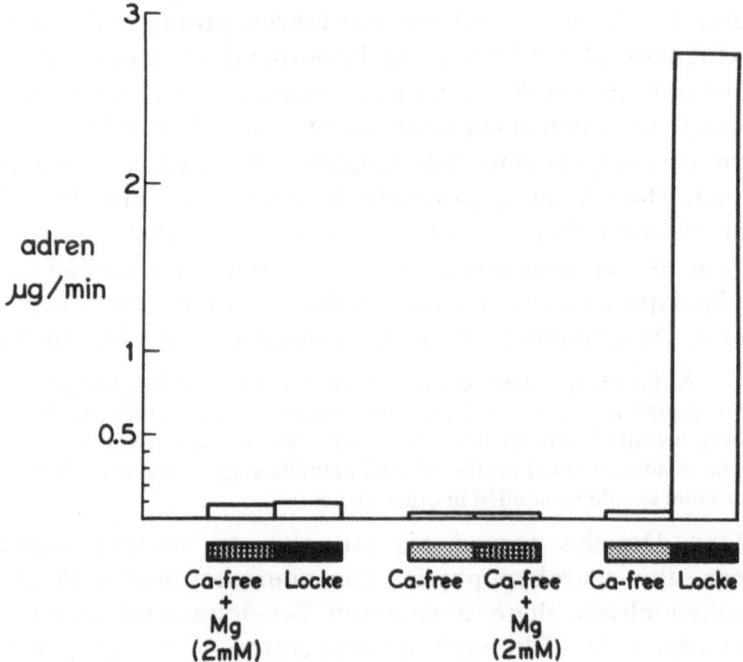

Fig. 4. The release of catecholamines from the cat adrenal gland by reintroducing calcium after perfusion with calcium-free solution, and the inhibition of this phenomenon by magnesium (Douglas and Rubin, 1963).

inhibits the secretory response to acetylcholine as well as to calcium. These results were compatible with the existing evidence concerning the mode of action of acetylcholine at other sites of cholinergic transmission where it was thought to act at the outer surface of the membrane to increase permeability.

The calcium dependence of acetylcholine in the secretory response might be explained by a need for calcium in the binding to receptors on the chromaffin cells, but this possibility was mitigated not only by the ability of calcium itself to elicit secretion but also by the finding that calcium is required for catecholamine secretion elicited by excess potassium, which presumably acts by depolarizing the cell membrane in the absence of any known drug–receptor interaction. Moreover, the adrenal medulla is stimulated by a large number of diverse chemical substances, and almost all of them require the presence of calcium for normal secretory activity. Thus the action of calcium on the medulla is thought to underlie a general mechanism whereby substances promote the inward movement of calcium by altering the permeability properties of the cell membrane. On the basis of these studies, calcium is viewed as the link in the chain of events initiated at the cell membrane by the action of acetylcholine that triggers the release of secretory product. This sequence, in which calcium is considered the prime agent, was described as "stimulus–secretion coupling."

The experiments on the adrenal medulla were viewed from a broad perspective, as evidenced by the following quotation from a paper by Douglas and Rubin in *The Journal of Physiology* in 1963:

> At the present time very little is known of the way in which glands are caused to secrete. Although the physiological secretogogues have been identified in many instances, their mode of action is still obscure. The results obtained on the adrenal medulla suggest that the effect of calcium should be studied in other glands.

And so Douglas turned his attention to another secretory system—the neurohypophysis. The neurosecretory cells of the neurohypophysis share a common developmental origin with chromaffin cells. Although neurosecretory cells are generally considered endocrine cells, they possess many of the morphological and electrophysiological features of conventional neurons. However, their axons do not synapse with other neurons or effector organs but release their product into the circulation. The synthesis and packaging of vasopressin and oxytocin into secretory granules with their binding protein, neurophysin, take place in the perikarya in the supraoptic–hypophyseal tracts of the hypothalamus, and the granules travel down the stalk to the nerve terminal by protoplasmic flow. Douglas, together with Alan Poisner and Ayako Ishida (Douglas and Poisner, 1964a,b; Douglas et al., 1965), carried out experiments on cut pieces of neurohypophysis to establish the calcium requirement for hormone release; they demonstrated that in this system, like the adrenal medulla, stimulation is associated with enhanced calcium entry. Stimulation of this preparation was generally elicited by excess potassium, although electric currents produce like effects. It is important to emphasize that here, as in the medulla, the actions of calcium were considered to be directly on the release process and not complicated by hormone synthesis, since neurosecretory terminals are unable to synthesize hormone.

The work of Douglas was not confined solely to secretory tissues of neurological ancestry but also extended to exocrine organs, for Douglas and Poisner also perfused the submaxillary salivary gland of the cat to study the influence of calcium on secretion (Douglas and Poisner, 1963). The salivary glands secrete water, electrolytes, and protein in response to stimulation of the parasympathetic (or sympathetic) nerves, and it was found that calcium deprivation produced a rapid diminution of protein secretion in response to acetylcholine but affected water and electrolyte secretion to a much lesser degree. The dissociation between the effects of acetylcholine on protein output on the one hand and water and electrolyte output on the other, in the absence of calcium, will be discussed later, but these experiments proved that the special function of calcium on the secretory process could be extended to include effects on a wide variety of secretory processes both neural and nonneural in origin.

Thus, based on the broad scope of his experiments, Douglas concluded that a similar process is at work in cells differing widely in the nature of their embryology, morphology, secretory product, and state of electrical excitability, and that the function of calcium in all of these systems is to participate in some key manner in the secretory process. He further observed that in all cells where a calcium-activated secretory mechanism had been demonstrated up to that time the secretory product was preformed and sequestered in membrane-bound granules (or vesicles), and he suggested that the function of calcium was to participate in a common mechanism for the extrusion of the contents of these granules. This concept is a very valid one, and more attention will be devoted to it in a subsequent chapter.

Following the reports of these studies, paper after paper began to appear in the scientific literature which implicated calcium in the secretion of a variety of different substances, which include norepinephrine from adrenergic nerves, insulin from the pancreatic cells, histamine and serotonin (5-HT) from mast cells and platelets, trophic hormones from the adenohypophysis, protein release from leukocytes and exocrine pancreas, hydrochloric acid and gastrin from the stomach, and other putative neurotransmitter substances such as γ-aminobutyric acid and glutamic acid. The ubiquitous involvement of calcium in the secretory mechanisms of such diverse organs would of course suggest that a common mechanism exists in which calcium plays a fundamental role. Therefore, before extending the scope of the discussion to other secretory organs it would seem to be worthwhile at this juncture to examine more closely the similarities and differences in the responsiveness of the cholinergic system, the neurohypophysis, and the adrenal medulla to a variety of conditions in order to ascertain whether the calcium requirement does indeed underlie a basically similar secretory mechanism.

Electrophysiological Events Associated with Secretion

Since the chromaffin cells, cholinergic neurons, and neurosecretory cells share a common origin in the neural crest, and are all derived from neuroblasts, it would be most reasonable to consider first the electrophysiological events associated with stimulation. Evidence obtained by Douglas and his colleagues established that the action of acetylcholine on adrenal chromaffin cells—similar to its action at other synaptic junctions where it plays the role of chemical transmitter—is associated with a depolarization of the plasma membrane and an increase in calcium entry (Douglas *et al.*, 1967b). Moreover, excess potassium depolarizes chromaffin cells *pari passu* with its secretory activity (Rubin and Miele, 1968), and with a given potassium concentration the secretory response can be correlated with the extracellular calcium concentration; in the absence of excess potassium, or any other stimulating agent, excess calcium is not sufficient to augment secretion. Such data suggest that permeability changes are necessary for the release reaction but they do not answer the question as to whether depolarization is a necessary step.

Early studies on the perfused adrenal showed that acetyl-choline remains an adequate stimulant even when perfusion is carried out with a sodium-free medium (Douglas and Rubin, 1961). Since sodium is the major extracellular cation and is therefore presumed to be responsible for carrying most of the inward current, depolarization would be severely impaired under these conditions, and indeed acetylcholine-induced depolarization of chromaffin cells is proportional to the concentration of external sodium (Douglas *et al.*, 1967b). Moreover, acetylcholine augments secretion in the presence of an excess of potassium (Douglas and Rubin, 1963), which would be expected to eradicate the disparity between the intracellular and extracellular potassium concentrations and therefore reduce the resting membrane potential to near zero. The stimulant activity of acetylcholine in the presence of excess potassium is manifest only in the presence of extracellular calcium. Thus it seems likely that under these conditions acetyl-choline acts not by depolarizing the cell but by directly enhancing calcium entry.

Additional information on the electrical events associated with the secretory events in the chromaffin cell was obtained with the use of local anesthetics. These agents were previously thought to inhibit generation of the action potential in excitable cells by inhibiting the sodium and potassium currents, although Feinstein (1964, 1966) had shown that local anesthetics inhibit calcium movement in smooth muscle and depress the phospholipid-facilitated transport of calcium from an aqueous phase into a lipid solvent phase. When tetracaine was added to the Locke's solution

perfusing the adrenal gland, the secretory response to acetylcholine and to potassium was inhibited (Rubin *et al.,* 1967).
Radiocalcium experiments showed that this inhibitory action was
the result of a blockade of calcium entry. Douglas and Kanno
(1967) further found that the addition of tetracaine to preparations of isolated chromaffin cells specifically blocked the inward
calcium current without affecting the inward sodium current;
conversely, tetrodotoxin, which blocks the inward sodium current,
does not inhibit the secretory response to calcium elicited by excess
potassium (Rubin and Jaanus, unpublished observations). Thus an
inhibition of depolarization *per se* is not sufficient to depress
secretion, but a blockade of the inward calcium current is required
in order to inhibit the release response. These experiments support
a scheme which describes stimulation of the chromaffin cell
membrane by acetylcholine as a permeability change in the
membrane allowing calcium to move down its concentration
gradient into the cell to reach the critical site to trigger the
secretory response. Calcium entry—and not depolarization *per
se*—is viewed as the key event (Rubin, 1970).

In cholinergic nerves the chemical transmitter, acetylcholine,
is stored in the nerve endings in cell organelles called vesicles. At
the neuromuscular junction the miniature end-plate potentials
(1–2 mV) are presumed to be a consequence of the spontaneous
release of quanta (or packets) of acetylcholine, since stimulation
with such agents as excess potassium increases the frequency of
these miniature potentials in a graded manner (Liley, 1956; Gage,
1967) (Fig. 5). It has been postulated that the nerve impulse
changes the permeability properties of the nerve terminal membrane to calcium, which causes an increase in the statistical
probability that interactions between vesicle and cell membrane
will occur, leading to augmented release (Katz, 1958, 1969). This
theory is based not only on the fact that electrical stimulation or
high potassium enhances calcium uptake into nerve preparations
but also on the close relationship between the extracellular calcium
concentration and the release reaction. Evoked acetylcholine
release is diminished or abolished by calcium deprivation, and the
amount of transmitter released depends on the extracellular
calcium concentration (cf. Rubin, 1970). This relationship be-

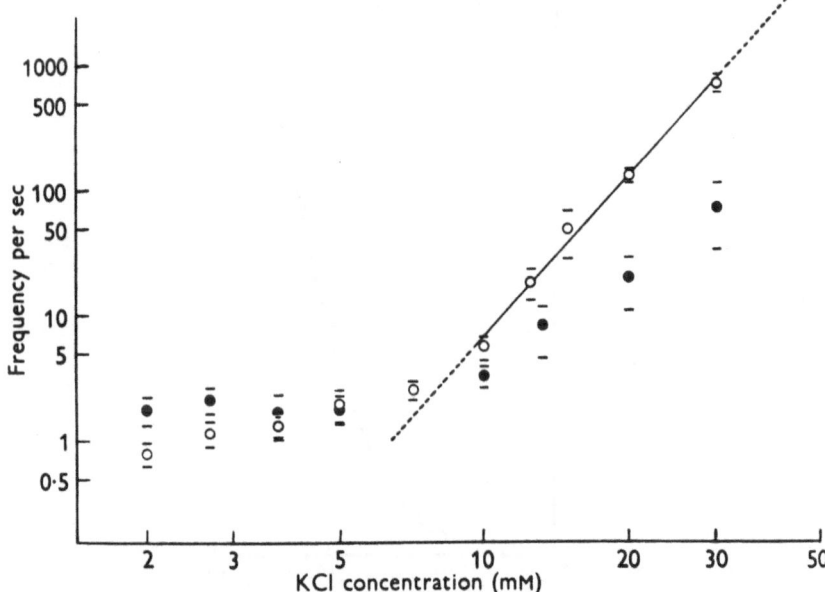

Fig. 5. Effect of potassium concentration on miniature end-plate potential frequency in the rat diaphragm myoneural preparation. Open and filled circles represent mean frequencies obtained with preparations bathed in normal calcium (2 mM) and 1 mM and 12.5 mM magnesium, respectively (Liley, 1956).

tween extracellular calcium and the release reaction is striking, as evidenced by the fact that within a certain concentration range (< 1 mM) a doubling of the calcium concentration increases the amplitude of the end-plate potential sixteenfold (Dodge and Rahamimoff, 1967; Rahamimoff, 1970) (Fig. 6). At calcium concentrations higher than about 10 mM, acetylcholine output no longer increases, and may even decrease, due to the membrane-stabilizing effects of calcium. The nonlinear relationship between the calcium concentration and acetylcholine release is in harmony with the suggestion originally proposed by del Castillo and Katz (1954) that calcium combines with a hypothetical receptor (X) on the membrahe surface of the nerve terminal and it is this reversible CaX complex which is responsible for the release reaction. Dodge and Rahamimoff (1967) have explained this nonlinear relationship by postulating that four CaX must act simultaneously for the release of each quantal packet of transmitter by the nerve impulse.

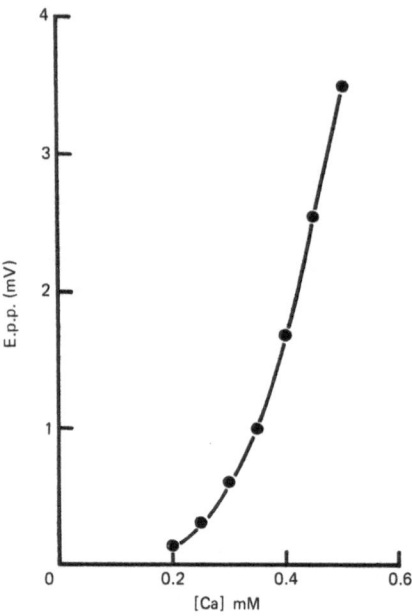

Fig. 6. Dependence of acetylcholine release from the frog sartorius myoneural junction on the external calcium concentration, as determined by the amplitude of the end-plate potential (Dodge and Rahamimoff, 1967).

Calcium entry during the arrival of the nerve impulse is an important event in the release reaction, but the question remains as to whether sodium entry is also a critical factor in coupling membrane depolarization to acetylcholine release. The early work of Hutter and Kostial (1955) showed that acetylcholine release from sympathetic ganglia elicited by electric current could be maintained during sodium deprivation as long as there was sufficient sodium (20%) to sustain impulse conduction. When the problem of impulse conduction was circumvented by the use of excess potassium to produce localized depolarization of the nerve endings, then acetylcholine release was observed in the complete absence of sodium as long as calcium was present. Katz and Miledi (1969) also demonstrated that sodium ions were not necessary for acetylcholine release from motor nerve endings by showing that in the complete absence of sodium, which should eliminate its regenerative influx, depolarizing pulses applied to the nerve terminals still produced enhanced release (Fig. 7). One might argue that there was enough residual sodium in the system to maintain depolarization of the nerve endings. However, this argument is nullified by the findings that tetrodotoxin completely blocks generation of the nerve impulse yet does not interfere with the release reaction, as evidenced by the fact that it does not change the size or frequency of the miniature end-plate potentials; and Katz and Miledi (1967a), employing a method of locally depolarizing the motor nerve ending in the presence of this poison, were able to demonstrate an increase in the quantal release of acetylcholine, as evidenced by the large end-plate potentials, as long as calcium was present in the bath.

The dissociation of the impulse-generating mechanism from the release mechanism indicates that the critical step involving the change in the resting membrane potential of the nerve ending is merely an opening of the gates to calcium ion. This concept is further supported by the finding that the ionophoretic application of calcium to the nerve ending must be accompanied by a depolarizing pulse in order to elicit a postsynaptic response (Katz

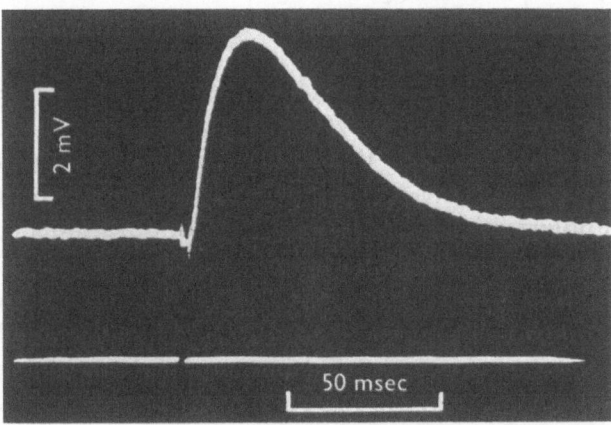

Fig. 7. End-plate potential recorded from the frog sartorius neuromuscular junction, evoked by focal depolarization of the nerve terminal after 6 hr exposure to isotonic calcium–Ringer (Katz and Miledi, 1969).

and Miledi, 1967b). Conversely, depolarizing current is not sufficient for inducing acetylcholine release unless it is preceded by a
calcium pulse.

Evidence adduced from studies on the neurohypophysis,
although not as comprehensive as that obtained on either the
adrenal medulla or cholinergic neuron, also strongly points to the
idea that calcium entry is the critical—and only required—ionic
event during membrane activation. Since the original work by
Douglas and Poisner (1946a, b), the importance of calcium for the
release of vasopressin and oxytocin from isolated rat
neurohypophyses has been clearly established. Release of
polypeptide hormone elicited by potassium or electric currents is
strongly dependent on the presence of calcium; output increases
with increasing concentrations up to 4 mM calcium; the observed
depression of secretion with higher calcium concentrations may be
ascribed to the stabilizing effects of calcium. Radiocalcium influx
and efflux are greatly augmented during exposure to excess
potassium, and although calcium uptake rises with the calcium
concentration, calcium uptake and hormonal secretion do not
parallel one another. Thus maximal uptake was obtained with
8.8 mM calcium, whereas maximal secretory activity occurred with
2–4 mM calcium. This suggests that under certain conditions much
more calcium enters the nerve terminals than that required to
produce the maximal response.

Whereas the evidence points to an important role for calcium
entry in vasopressin and oxytocin release, there is little or no
evidence in this system for the idea that the inward movement of
sodium ions is directly involved in the release of hormone. A
graded depolarization by excess potassium does indeed induce a
proportional enhancement of polypeptide hormone from the
isolated neurohypophysis in a manner analogous to that observed
for chromaffin tissue and cholinergic nerves. However, hormone
release in response to local depolarization of the nerve endings by
either potassium or electric current is not depressed in a sodium-
free medium but may even be enhanced (Douglas and Poisner,
1964a; Douglas and Sorimachi, 1971); moreover, the effective-
ness of excess potassium in eliciting graded secretory responses in
tetrodotoxin-treated lobes (Dreifuss et al., 1971) suggests that the

membrane and ionic events associated with the release of pituitary hormones closely resemble those in the adrenal chromaffin cells and at chemical synapses. These data from three different secretory systems lead to the irrefutable conclusion that the entry of calcium into the cell, and not depolarization, is the key ionic event in stimulus–secretion coupling, and activation of the cell membrane will lead to an enhanced release only when calcium can penetrate into the cell.

Role of Monovalent Cations

Although electrophysiological events produced by sodium ions do not appear to be directly involved in the entry of calcium into the cell, the intracellular concentration of sodium ions appears to indirectly affect the amount of secretory product released, especially under conditions of prolonged stimulation. Early experiments with the perfused cat adrenal showed that although acute sodium deprivation was associated with increased secretory responses, prolonged exposure to sodium-free solutions led to a deterioration of the release response (Douglas and Rubin, 1961). Banks (1970) later demonstrated that the secretory response of the perfused bovine adrenal may fall some 15 min after the onset of perfusion with a sodium-deficient solution, and he concluded that the decline was probably the result of a fall in the intracellular concentration of sodium. Further experimentation led him to the conclusion that the intracellular concentration of sodium is an important factor in controlling the entry of calcium into chromaffin cells.

The use of ouabain, a cardiac glycoside, has also contributed greatly to our understanding of the relative importance of calcium and sodium in the release process. Ouabain enhances the release of adrenal catecholamines in a calcium-dependent manner (Banks, 1967). The primary pharmacological action of the cardiac glycosides involves an inhibition of the enzyme system known as "Na−K+-dependent ATPase," which is closely associated with the transport of sodium and potassium ions across cell membranes and is responsible for maintaining the low levels of sodium and potassium in intra- and extracellular fluids, respectively. Thus the action of ouabain should be associated with a cellular accumulation of sodium, and indeed the medullary secretory activity of ouabain is blocked in a sodium-free solution, confirming that intracellular sodium is somehow involved in the calcium-dependent secretory process of the adrenal medulla (Banks, 1970).

The sodium concentration also affects the release of acetylcholine liberated by the nerve impulse. With low calcium concentrations, a sodium–calcium antagonism can be observed at the neuromuscular junction. When the extracellular calcium concentration is low, a decrease in the sodium concentration produces an increase in the quantal content, but when the calcium content is normal the same decrease in sodium concentration produces less marked changes (Kelly, 1969). Such findings suggest that calcium and sodium compete for a common site in the process of transmitter release. More quantitative studies by Colomo and Rahamimoff (1968) indicate that even in the normal ionic environment sodium ions do play a regulatory role in the release mechanism by competing with calcium (and magnesium) for vacated sites. Birks and Cohen (1968) also obtained indirect evidence that intracellular sodium affects acetylcholine release by showing that cardiac glycosides increase spontaneous and evoked release of transmitter from motor nerve terminals; these effects were slowed by sodium deprivation, suggesting that the effects produced by the glycosides were generated by an inhibition of the sodium pump and a resulting accumulation of sodium.

The relative expendability of sodium in the release process of the neurohypophysis has also been alluded to, as evidenced by Douglas and Poisner's (1964a) finding that striking secretory responses were still obtained in a sodium-free environment. However, ouabain—like potassium and electric currents—triggers polypeptide release from isolated rat neurohypophyses; this enhanced release depends on the presence of calcium and is associated with an increase in the sodium content of the glands (Dicker, 1966). So in this system—like the adrenal medulla and cholinergic nerve endings—sodium appears to be indirectly involved in the release process by modulating the distribution of calcium.

The indirect role of cellular sodium in the secretory process can be explained on the basis of its interaction with the key cation, calcium. Baker and his colleagues showed that in the crustacean neuron calcium influx increases strikingly when the external sodium is removed or when the internal sodium concentration is raised (cf. Baker, 1972). These findings explain the enhanced release observed during brief exposures to sodium-free solutions and the effect of cardiac glycosides on the basis of an increase in calcium accumulation in the cytoplasm—the former situation the result of calcium displacing sodium from sites associated with entry, the latter situation explained by a rise in cellular sodium which is exchanged for extracellular calcium. Conversely, then, a lowering of the internal sodium concentration causes a decrease in calcium influx, which would explain the inability to maintain secretory responses after prolonged sodium deprivation.

The enhancement of calcium entry after a reduction in external sodium is not restricted to secretory organs but has been demonstrated in a variety of other tissues, such as skeletal, cardiac, and smooth muscle preparations, and in liver (cf. Baker, 1972). Niedergerke (1963) suggested that in heart muscle the carrier molecule for which sodium and calcium compete is negatively charged, so that it moves inward when the membrane is depolarized. A similar mechanism may account for the increase in the secretory response after stimulation, which results in an increase in the concentration of CaX at the surface of the membrane. The relationship between calcium uptake and the sodium concentration of cells was very clearly defined by Cooke and Robinson (1971), who showed that the ouabain-induced increase of radiocalcium and sodium in brain slices was blocked by tetrodotoxin, although, in the absence of ouabain, toxin blocked sodium accumulation but had no discernible effect on calcium accumulation. These data indicate that the effect of ouabain on calcium flux is mediated through its effect on sodium movements.

The conclusion which thus emerges is that the intracellular level of calcium—which is critical for activating the release reaction—is determined by the electrochemical gradient for sodium. It will be seen that ouabain can act as a secretogogue in other calcium-dependent secretory systems—most notably, the insulin-secreting pancreatic islet cells—and the effects of the glycoside result from an inhibition of the sodium pump because they are not demonstrable in the absence of external sodium. The secretory activity of ouabain can be mimicked by potassium deprivation, since this monovalent cation is required for optimal ATPase activity to drive the sodium pump. Thus it appears that any situation which affects the cellular level of sodium will, in turn, affect the rate of calcium influx and thereby influence secretory activity.

Multivalent Cations

A clue to the nature of the role of calcium in the secretory process may be found in the relative activities of other divalent cations on the secretory process, which would provide information on the calcium-receptive process. For example, is the property exhibited by calcium only a matter of charge and will other divalent cations also act in a similar manner to calcium? Indeed, in some biological processes the role of calcium is relatively unspecific and a number of divalent cations can substitute for calcium; this appears to be the situation in regard to the effects of calcium on permeability properties of tissue. Such a comparative study of the effects of other alkaline earth metals on the release mechanism was made very early in this century by Mines (1911), who found that both strontium and barium, but not magnesium, could replace calcium in maintaining neuromuscular transmission, and he suggested that it is not their electrical charge but some special chemical property that enables these cations to combine with certain tissue constituents in a manner in which magnesium cannot. The more detailed consideration of existing evidence which follows generally bears out Mines's conclusions.

Strontium. Strontium appears to be an effective substitute for calcium in almost all aspects of the secretory process. When strontium ions are substituted for calcium, the release of acetylcholine from motor nerve endings has properties similar to release with calcium. Thus in the presence of strontium, release is quantal in nature, and typical fluctuations in the amplitude of the end-plate potential appear which are predicted accurately by the Poisson theorem (Dodge *et al.*, 1969). Although activation of neurotransmitter release by calcium and strontium is qualitatively similar, there are quantitative differences, in the sense that strontium is much less effective than calcium. Thus 2.0 mM strontium gives transmitter release approximately equal to that of 0.3 mM calcium. This large disparity in the potency of these two alkaline earths is not due to a difference in the affinity for the hypothetical sites X, but appears related to their relative efficacy in directly activating the release process (Rahamimoff, 1970).

In the adrenal medulla, strontium also acts like calcium, since it evokes catecholamine secretion when added after a period of calcium deprivation (in the absence of magnesium) or during exposure to acetylcholine or excess potassium (Douglas and Rubin, 1964a). Also, although excess strontium is without a stimulant effect when added during perfusion with normal media, it potentiates secretory responses to acetylcholine or potassium just as does excess calcium. All of these procedures probably increase the permeability of the chromaffin cell membrane and allow strontium to penetrate the cell membrane. Strontium can also substitute for calcium in preventing this permeability change from occurring in cells perfused with calcium-free solution, so that its action on the permeability properties of chromaffin cells resembles that of calcium. It should be emphasized that the effects of strontium are due to its intrinsic ability to activate the secretory mechanism and not to an indirect effect by releasing a bound form of cellular calcium (Douglas and Rubin, 1964a). This possibility had to be ruled out because such a mechanism may be responsible for the activity of strontium and other cations which can substitute for calcium in maintaining contraction of skeletal muscle (Frank, 1962).

Barium.   Barium, a divalent cation closely related to calcium and strontium, also influences acetylcholine release from cholinergic nerves. The effect of barium at the superior cervical ganglion resembles calcium in that when added to the calcium-free perfusion solution it restores acetylcholine output, and when added to calcium-containing media it augments acetylcholine release (Douglas *et al.*, 1961). Since barium can penetrate axons during stimulation, it appears that conditions which increase barium ions within the cell will trigger release just as does calcium accumulation.

In the adrenal medulla, barium can also activate the calcium-dependent process involved in the secretion of catecholamines (Douglas and Rubin, 1964b). Like calcium (and strontium), barium can evoke secretion when introduced after perfusion with calcium-free solution and maintain the secretory responses to acetylcholine or potassium which would otherwise be absent in the calcium-deprived medium. However, barium differs from calcium and strontium in that it stimulates catecholamine secretion without an associated increase in cell permeability produced by acetylcholine, excess potassium, or calcium deprivation. The stimulant effect of barium is mediated through a depolarization of the chromaffin cells, and its activity as a secretogogue is blocked by magnesium; however, the role of calcium in the stimulant action of barium is unusual in the sense that it inhibits barium-evoked secretion. Thus barium may act to alter cell permeability by displacing a critical calcium fraction from the plasma membrane.

Barium also greatly potentiates vasopressin output from isolated rat neurohypophyses just as it potentiates acetylcholine release from cholinergic nerve endings, and increases spontaneous release of vasopressin just as it enhances spontaneous catecholamine secretion from medullary chromaffin cells (Dicker, 1966). Moreover, in very low concentrations (2.5 μM) barium maintains the increase in vasopressin and oxytocin release usually observed with excess potassium in the presence of calcium. It thus appears that barium, once inside the cell, mimics the action of calcium on the secretory process, but its effects on the membrane properties of secretory cells differ in some ways from those of calcium and more closely resemble the depolarizing effects of potassium.

Magnesium. The ability of strontium and barium to substitute for calcium in the secretory process is not simply due to the fact that they are divalent cations; magnesium, though having chemical properties similar to calcium, antagonizes the actions of calcium in many biological systems (Engbaek, 1952) and depresses acetylcholine output from preganglionic sympathetic nerves

(Hutter and Kostial, 1954). The competitive nature of this antagonism is demonstrated by the fact that high calcium relieves the magnesium block (Fig. 8). Magnesium also inhibits the release of acetylcholine from motor nerve terminals, as evidenced by the finding of del Castillo and Katz (1954) that a nerve impulse releases more acetylcholine if external calcium is increased (within limits) or if magnesium is lowered. In discussing this antagonism, they suggested that calcium and magnesium compete for the hypothetical carrier molecule X. Jenkinson (1957) obtained quantitative data on acetylcholine release (as measured by the amplitude of the end-plate potential) over a wide range of calcium and magnesium concentrations, and his data were in harmony with the hypothesis that these ions compete for receptor molecules which control the amount of transmitter released by a nerve impulse. There is thus convincing evidence that magnesium blocks transmitter release by competing with calcium for critical binding sites on the nerve terminal membrane, but it has not been ascertained whether the antagonism occurs on the outer or inner surface of the presynaptic membrane. However, the ability of excess magnesium to reduce calcium entry into nerve preparations after electrical stimulation (Blaustein, 1971) or high potassium (Lipicky *et al.*,

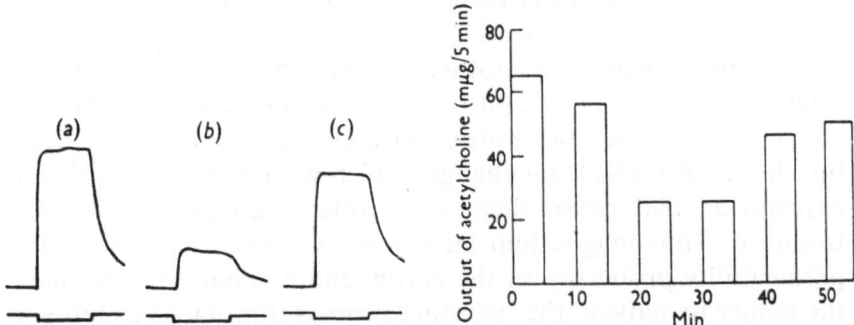

Fig. 8. The inhibitory effect of magnesium on ganglionic transmission and its reversal by excess calcium. The preganglionic cervical sympathetic nerve of the cat was stimulated and contractions of the nictitating membrane were recorded. The ganglion was perfused with (a) normal Locke's solution, (b) Locke's solution plus 20 mM MgCl₂, and (c) Locke's solution used in (b) plus 4.2 mM CaCl₂. The vertical bars represent the amount of acetylcholine released by nerve stimulation. After sample 2, 15 mM MgCl₂ was added, and after 4, 4.2 mM CaCl₂ was added (Hutter and Kostial, 1954).

1963) suggests a competition for sites involved with permeation of the plasma membranes; in fact, kinetic data indicate that magnesium competes with calcium at the same site as sodium (Colomo and Rahamimoff, 1968).

The action of magnesium on the secretory response of the adrenal medulla is also inhibitory (Douglas and Rubin, 1961, 1963), and it has been employed to provide evidence for the concept that calcium entry provides the key link in "stimulus–secretion coupling." Thus magnesium, a competitive inhibitor of medullary secretion, markedly depresses calcium exchange between the gland and the perfusate (Rubin *et al.*, 1967). The effect of magnesium on medullary chromaffin cells may also be simplistically explained by the concept that magnesium competes with calcium for transport sites and the entry of magnesium into the cell is not associated with catecholamine secretion. And indeed magnesium, even in concentrations as high as 80 mM, is not able to replace calcium as a coupling agent. On the other hand, there is evidence to suggest that during stimulation magnesium does not penetrate chromaffin cells as freely as calcium, since calcium supports the acetylcholine-induced depolarization of isolated chromaffin cells in the absence of sodium, whereas the depolarization in response to acetylcholine does not increase as the magnesium concentration is raised (Douglas *et al.*, 1967b).

Magnesium also has another action on the chromaffin cells not related to a direct action on the secretory process but related to effects on the permeability properties. That is, magnesium protects the chromaffin cells from changes which usually occur on calcium deprivation and cause them to secrete when calcium is reintroduced. Thus magnesium mimics the action of calcium on the permeability properties of the chromaffin cell but does not have the ability to activate the secretory process (Fig. 4). The ability of magnesium to mimic the effects of calcium on regulating cell permeability may also explain why magnesium and calcium exert synergistic effects on electrical properties of excitable tissues, although magnesium antagonizes the effect of calcium on neurotransmitter release.

The calcium-entry hypothesis also gains support from the experiments with magnesium on the neurohypophysis, where the calcium-dependent evoked release of vasopressin and oxytocin is inhibited by excess magnesium (Douglas and Poisner, 1964a). Although the enhanced calcium uptake associated with stimulation is depressed by magnesium (Douglas and Poisner, 1964b), high magnesium inhibits calcium uptake by only 30% but blocks secretion by 70–80%. This suggests that at least some of the effects of magnesium may be produced not only by affecting the uptake of calcium into the cell but also by interacting with calcium in the interior of the cell. The interaction between calcium and magnesium at presynaptic motor nerve endings may also occur at more than one site (Cooke *et al.*, 1973).

Manganese. In addition to magnesium there are other cations which inhibit the release process and are known inhibitors of calcium movements across cell membranes. Manganese exerts inhibitory effects on the neuromuscular junction which are qualitatively similar to magnesium, but it is about twenty times more potent (Meiri and Rahamimoff, 1972). With the addition of a "competitive" ion such as manganese, depolarization becomes less capable of accelerating the miniature end-plate potentials above their resting frequency. The action of manganese is believed to be on the influx of calcium ions, for manganese had been found to act as an antagonist to calcium in many biological processes (Fatt and Ginsborg, 1958; Hagiwara and Nakajima, 1966). Moreover, the influx of calcium ions into nerve fibers which occurs after depolarization can be divided into two distinct components: an early phase that can be suppressed by tetrodotoxin and a later phase that can be blocked by manganese or magnesium ions (Baker, 1972); it is this late calcium flux which is presumably associated with transmitter release.

Lanthanum. The trivalent cation lanthanum is also a potent inhibitor of calcium transport in a variety of membrane systems, since it inhibits calcium transport in mitochondria (Mela, 1969) and muscle preparations (Langer and Frank, 1972) and inhibits calcium spikes recorded from crustacean muscle fibers (Hagiwara and Takahashi, 1967); so it is not surprising to find that lanthanum is a very potent inhibitor of neurally evoked acetylcholine release from motor nerve endings (DeBassio *et al.*, 1971; Miledi, 1971). The ability of lanthanum to decrease the probability of release by depressing the inward calcium current responsible for triggering the secretory process is supported by Miledi's demonstration that lanthanum blocks the tetrodotoxin-insensitive calcium current in the presynaptic nerve terminal at the squid giant synapse (Miledi, 1971). Lanthanum is also a potent stabilizer of cell membranes, so that part of the action of this cation may be to resist the change in the resting membrane potential after stimulation (Takata et al., 1966; Blaustein and Goldman, 1968). However, it should be emphasized that lanthanum does not inhibit release by decreasing the size of the action potential, since in the presence of lanthanum nerve impulses continue to invade the nerve terminal but are unable to release transmitter (Miledi, 1971).

Since the crystal ionic radii of lanthanum and calcium are similar, they might be expected to compete for the same negatively charged membrane sites; however, lanthanum, having a higher valency, will have a greater affinity for these sites. The result will be a hyperstabilization of the membrane and a decreased cellular uptake of calcium. The ability of lanthanum to hyperstabilize the membrane as well as prevent calcium flux (Weiss and Goodman, 1969) may explain why in the adrenal medulla lanthanum so profoundly inhibits the secretory response to acetylcholine (Borowitz, 1972).

Lanthanum can also increase spontaneous release of neurotransmitter (DeBassio et al., 1971) and medullary catecholamine (Borowitz, 1972). The increase in transmitter release is eventually associated with complete depletion of synaptic vesicles (Heuser and Miledi, 1971). A search for an explanation for this phenomenon leads us to the most likely conclusion that lanthanum, although distributed mainly through the extracellular spaces, can gain access to intracellular sites and will enhance secretion by causing the accumulation of free calcium in the cytoplasm by inhibiting its sequestration by intracellular organelles such as mitochondria.

Conclusions

Under certain unusual conditions, secretion can continue, to some degree at least, after calcium deprivation. Thus an increase in osmotic pressure, black-widow spider venom, and ethanol all cause an increase in the frequency of miniature end-plate potentials which is independent of the external calcium concentration (Quastel *et al.*, 1971). The increase in spontaneous catecholamine output engendered by severe sodium deprivation is also unaffected by perfusion with calcium-free media (Douglas and Rubin, 1963), and, finally, enhanced secretion of vasopressin produced by sulfhydryl inhibitors or cooling not only can occur in the absence of calcium but also appears to be unaffected by a variety of changes in the ionic milieu, such as excess magnesium or potassium (Douglas and Ishida, 1965; Douglas *et al.*, 1965). These studies are of interest, since they do show that under unusual circumstances hormone release can still occur in the absence of extracellular calcium.

However, it is difficult to explain these stimulant actions within the scope of physiological mechanisms, for when release is elicited by electric currents or by physiological transmitter the importance of calcium becomes readily manifest. It thus seems fair to conclude that calcium is the physiological coupling agent between the excitatory and secretory processes of the adrenal chromaffin cell, cholinergic nerve ending, and neurohypophyseal–neurosecretory cell. Moreover, the calcium-receptive mechanism in each of these systems is similar in its responsiveness to the various alkaline earth metals. Thus each responds not only to calcium but also to strontium and barium, but is inhibited by magnesium. Sodium plays no direct role in any of these secretory organs, except that its presence in the extra- and intracellular fluids is important for controlling calcium levels in the cells. These data indicate that although there may be minor differences from one system to another, a basically similar process underlies the secretory mechanisms in these three somewhat diverse systems. It would not be premature at this point to note that the effects of cations on the secretory process are remarkably similar to their effects on muscle contraction; it enables one to begin to draw parallels between the processes of "stimulus–secretion coupling" and "excitation–contraction coupling."

OTHER NEURONAL SYSTEMS

Although the evidence adduced up to now may tempt one to infer that calcium plays a general role in the events by which activation of the neuronal membrane is coupled to the secretory process, other examples of a similar calcium action are required in order to fortify the assumption that this represents a general phenomenon rather than mere examples of a specific interaction of calcium with isolated events in certain individual secretory systems. There is no problem in finding such examples, for the importance of calcium in synaptic transmission has been established in most systems where such studies have been carried out.

Excitatory and Inhibitory Synapses

Calcium ions can affect the release from nerve tissue of putative transmitter substances, including dopamine (Bustos and Roth, 1972), γ-aminobutyric acid (Otsuka et al., 1966), and glutamate (Usherwood et al., 1968), as well as acetylcholine and norepinephrine. Chemically mediated synaptic transmission —whether it is excitatory or inhibitory—depends on the presence of calcium in the extracellular fluid. At the inhibitory synapses of the neuromuscular junction of the lobster, where evidence indicates that γ-aminobutyric acid may be the chemical transmitter agent, nerve stimulation in low-calcium media fails to produce inhibitory junctional potentials and release of γ-aminobutyric acid despite the recording of normal action potentials from the nerve (Otsuka et al., 1966).

This fundamental effect of calcium on synaptic transmission has been demonstrated not only on peripheral neurons but also on nerve tissue of the central nervous system (cf. Rubin, 1970); it also extends down through the phylogenetic scale to invertebrate systems, such as arthropod and crustacean nerve terminals (Hoyle, 1955; Berlind and Cooke, 1971). Thus l-glutamate, and not acetylcholine, is considered to be the putative excitatory transmitter released from insect and crustacean motor nerve terminals, and in these systems calcium ions are essential for the development of junctional potentials (Usherwood et al., 1968; Bracho and Orkand, 1970). Furthermore, the release of transmitter appears to be proportional to the external calcium concentration and is antagonized by magnesium. The importance of calcium in neurotransmitter release is so well defined that during calcium deprivation one may correlate the decrease in the physiological response with the decrease in the release of the putative chemical transmitter, and thereby provide further evidence that the substance is indeed the chemical transmitter agent at that site.

We have previously considered the work of Katz and his associates on the neuromuscular junction, and that carried out at sympathetic ganglia, which demonstrated the critical role of calcium in transmitter release at cholinergic junctions. However, over the years a controversy had raged over how calcium deprivation depresses transmitter release. At cholinergic synapses it had been established that a decrease in the external calcium concentration leads to a decrease in the amount of transmitter released by the nerve impulse. However, since it was also known that prolonged calcium lack renders nerve fibers inexcitable, it could have been concluded that the depression of transmitter release is merely a consequence of a lack of invasion of the nerve terminal by the impulse. Katz and Miledi (cf. Katz, 1969), in a series of very elegant experiments, ascertained that this latter alternative was not a valid one, but that calcium acts directly on the process that leads to transmitter release. Although the experiments, which shall be briefly described, were also carried out on the frog neuromuscular junction, perhaps the more definitive experiments were conducted at neuroneuronal synapse of squid stellate ganglion. In this invertebrate junction, where there are both excitatory and inhibitory synapses, transmission is effected by the release of transmitter(s) whose identity is still unknown, although there is some evidence to suggest that it may be glutamate. Moreover, the ion fluxes involved in transmitter release are also not well understood.

Katz and Miledi (cf. Katz, 1969) perceived that the giant squid synapse—because of its large size—would permit insertion of microelectrodes in both the pre- and postsynaptic elements, and in this preparation they clearly demonstrated that in low calcium the nerve impulse still reaches the nerve ending but does not evoke a postsynaptic potential. This critical finding established that the effects of calcium deprivation are not attributable to actions on the electrical properties of the neuronal elements, but to a direct action on the release of transmitter. With this same preparation, Miledi and Slater (1966) showed that in low-calcium solutions transmission could be restored by *extracellular* ionophoretic application to a localized area of the presynaptic nerve endings. The lack of action of calcium, when injected *inside* the presynaptic terminal, suggests that the reaction which leads to transmitter release requires the combination of calcium with a membrane component accessible only from the outside of the membrane.

Adrenergic Synapses

The importance of selecting an appropriate biological system and adopting the proper experimental conditions to test a hypothesis has already been alluded to, and with the idea of reinforcing this important concept as background let us now consider the role of calcium in the release of catecholamine from adrenergic nerve terminals in peripheral effector organs. The effects of calcium on the release of norepinephrine by sympathetic nerve endings have been studied by many different workers using a variety of isolated organ preparations. The release of neurotransmitter from adrenergic synapses, as from cholinergic synapses, can be studied either by perfusing the organ with a saline medium and assaying the effluent after stimulation or by measuring the response of the end organ after electrical or chemical stimulation of the nerve. The former procedure is obviously preferable, since the transmitter output can be determined directly.

Hukovic and Muscholl (1962) were the first to demonstrate the critical role of calcium in the release of catecholamine from adrenergic nerves. They showed that the release of norepinephrine from the rabbit heart induced by electrical stimulation of the cardiac accelerator nerves was drastically reduced after perfusion with calcium-deficient solutions. Other evidence to support this postulated role of calcium has been obtained using the guinea pig vas deferens and heart, cat spleen and iris, and rabbit colon, ileum, and ear artery preparations (cf. Rubin, 1970; Smith and Winkler, 1972). And there is no doubt that all of these studies have established a basic similarity between the release of catecholamines from the adrenal medulla and the release of norepinephrine from postganglionic sympathetic fibers. Thus norepinephrine output induced by nerve stimulation varies directly with the calcium concentration of the medium (Fig. 9), magnesium antagonizes evoked release, and barium and strontium substitute for calcium in the release process (Bouillin, 1967; Kirpekar and Misu, 1967).

Yet, although it is generally agreed that calcium is required for norepinephrine release from adrenergic nerve endings, there are other events that take place in the adrenergic nerve during transmitter release which make it difficult to interpret precisely how various cations and other chemical substances interact in the events following nerve stimulation. As in other neurons, electrical stimulation of the adrenergic nerve initiates action potentials conducted along the axon to the nerve terminal, and depolarization of the nerve terminal causes release of norepinephrine by promoting the entry of calcium. This raises the question as to whether a given substance may enhance or inhibit norepinephrine release directly by affecting calcium entry or indirectly by affecting the electrical properties of the nerve. For example, it is known that tetraethylammonium enhances norepinephrine release, but it is not clear whether it does so directly by facilitating the entry of calcium or indirectly by prolonging the duration of the action

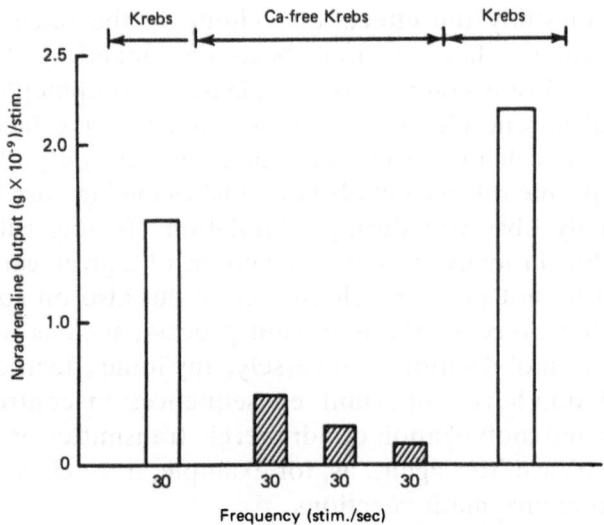

Fig. 9. The effect of calcium omission on norepinephrine output from the perfused cat spleen following nerve stimulation (Kirpekar and Misu, 1967).

potential as the result of its ability to specifically block the outward potassium current (Kirpekar *et al.*, 1972). Conversely, local anesthetic agents may depress release by inhibiting membrane depolarization or inhibiting the subsequent influx of calcium. Another complication is the fact that output of norepinephrine represents the amount of amine initially released minus the amount that is taken back by an active reuptake mechanism in the adrenergic neurons which conserves catecholamines and terminates their actions. Since a cation dependence of catecholamine uptake exists in adrenergic effector organs (Blaszkowski and Bogdanski, 1971; Nash *et al.*, 1972), a block of the reuptake mechanism—as well as a direct effect on the release process—could account for increased amounts of norepinephrine retrieved.

Also, unlike the adrenal medulla, the peripheral stores of catecholamine are rapidly turning over, so that while norepinephrine is being released from nerve endings, under the proper conditions new transmitter is being synthesized and incorporated into storage vesicles prior to release. Since sodium, for example, is required for storage as well as uptake of norepinephrine in nerve terminals (Blaszkowski and Bogdanski, 1971), it is apparent that one cannot study the effects of sodium on the release process without other related actions becoming manifest. Moreover, synthesis is closely coupled to the release of norepinephrine from peripheral adrenergic nerves, as evidenced by the fact that the removal of calcium from the medium not only diminishes norepinephrine release but also diminishes the increase in synthesis normally observed during stimulation (Boadle-Biber *et al.*, 1970). Thus in many systems the actions of a given cation might very well be not only on release *per se* but also on some other process that precedes the extrusion process, such as transmitter synthesis or mobilization. Conversely, any ionic effects on release can, and do, have important consequences in controlling the synthesis and mobilization of adrenergic transmitter or any other chemical transmitter agent, as, for example, through end-product inhibition of enzymatic reactions.

Another problem associated with the study of the release mechanism from adrenergic nerves, as well as other neuronal structures, is that not only do they respond to electrical stimulation but they may also respond to chemical stimulation; and there is much evidence to indicate that pharmacological release may depend on an entirely different mechanism from physiological release. Thus we have previously discussed the fact that although transmitter release from the neuromuscular junction elicited by nerve stimulation is closely related to the calcium concentration of the medium, the augmented release of transmitter induced by black-widow spider venom and by ethanol—as measured by the increased frequency of the miniature end-plate potential—is the same in calcium-free media as when calcium is present (Longenecker *et al.*, 1970; Quastel *et al.*, 1971). Similarly, the release of norepinephrine from peripheral adrenergic organs by the indirectly acting sympathomimetic amine, tyramine, appears to occur through a nonphysiological mechanism not dependent on the presence of calcium (Thoenen *et al.*, 1969; Chubb *et al.*, 1972). The calcium requirement for norepinephrine release induced by electric current can even be bypassed if a high enough current strength is utilized (Katz and Kopin, 1969a). That all gradations of the calcium requirement exist is also well exemplified by the work of Kopin and his associates, who showed that while the release of norepinephrine from brain slices induced by electrical stimulation requires calcium, the release of 5-hydroxytryptamine is unaffected by calcium deprivation under similar conditions (Katz and Kopin, 1969b).

All of these data may indicate that calcium is not completely essential to the final steps by which norepinephrine, or any other transmitter agent, is released. However, the lack of calcium dependence with a given stimulus must be ascertained by careful experimentation. There is little doubt that different agents in varying concentrations show a differential sensitivity to calcium deprivation, so that care must be taken to ascertain that a system is indeed calcium deprived, and various concentrations of the stimulant—whether electrical or chemical—must be employed, because supramaximal stimulation can at times activate the release mechanism in the absence of calcium (cf. Schneider, 1972; Ziance *et al.*, 1972). Although it may very well be that certain secretory systems can operate in the absence of calcium, one may also argue that secretory responses observed during calcium deprivation are due to persisting extracellular calcium or to some nonextractable calcium stores. An active role for a tightly bound cellular calcium pool would imply that stimulating agents, especially in high concentrations, can act directly on cellular calcium-storing structures to release calcium without necessarily altering the permeability properties of the plasma membrane and thereby circumvent the requirement for a more labile pool of calcium. However, this speculation, unfortunately, still does not provide us with a clear and simple explanation of the factors responsible for the differential sensitivity of secretory systems to calcium deprivation, and it will be interesting to see how this problem is eventually solved.

RELEASE OF OTHER BIOGENIC AMINES

Histamine

In addition to catecholamines, histamine and 5-hydroxytryptamine (serotonin) are two other biogenic amines stored and released from a variety of tissues as the result of their sequestration in mast cells, leukocytes, and blood platelets. The histamine present in mast cells is stored in membrane-bound cellular organelles, and all of the available evidence favors the hypothesis that histamine release from mast cells occurs by expulsion of the granular material through the cell membrane. This observed process in mast cells has been termed degranulation and appears to correspond to exocytosis in endocrine secretory systems (Röhlich et al., 1971). However, since degranulation has been observed only in in vitro systems, nothing definite can as yet be concluded as to whether the same factors regulate histamine release from mast cells in vivo.

The physiological stimulus for the release of histamine is the antigen–antibody reaction, although a variety of other diverse substances are able to stimulate histamine release, such as organic bases (48/80), bee venom, Ascaris extract, and ATP (Uvnäs, 1964). Here again, as in the secretory systems discussed previously which store secretory product within granules, there appears to be the same common denominator in the release process, namely the requirement for calcium.

It was in 1958 that Mongar and Schild published their now classical paper on the effect of calcium on the anaphylactic release of histamine from sensitized guinea pig lung. They demonstrated that the release of histamine induced by anaphylaxis was markedly inhibited by calcium lack (Fig. 10), but neither potassium nor sodium was an essential requirement; in fact, a substantial amount of histamine release was obtained in a sucrose solution which contained only calcium chloride and a trace of potassium bicarbonate. Of further interest was the observation that the inhibitory effect of calcium deprivation was overcome by an increase in pH, which suggested to Mongar and Schild that the anaphylactic reaction requires bound calcium and that the binding decreases with a fall in pH. The requirement for a bound fraction of calcium may explain why in certain histamine-releasing systems and under certain conditions it can be difficult to demonstrate the requirement for calcium.

Since Mongar and Schild also found that the inhibition of histamine release was not accompanied by any change in oxygen

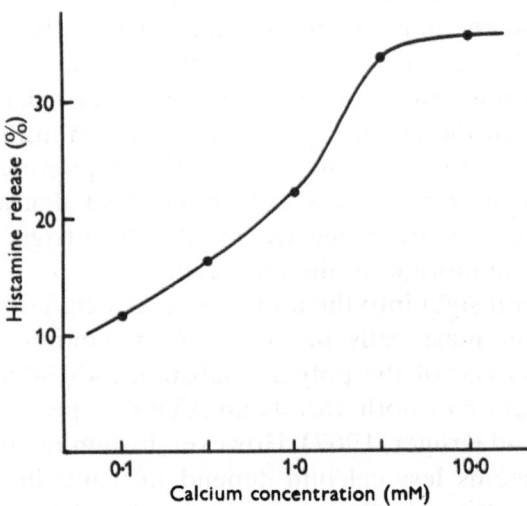

Fig. 10. The effect of calcium on antigen-induced histamine release from chopped sensitized guinea pig lung bathed in isotonic saline solution (Mongar and Schild, 1958).

consumption, they concluded that the effect of calcium deprivation was not related to a calcium action on energy metabolism. They ascribed the sequence of calcium-dependent events in histamine release analogous to the fixation of complement by antigen–antibody complex, and they viewed the action of calcium as an activation of an unstable enzyme system involved in the process of histamine release. Envisaging the sequence of events of release in terms of a complement fixation reaction loses some support in light of the fact that although calcium potentiates the complement fixation reaction, strontium and barium cannot re-store complement fixation in the absence of calcium but are able to replace calcium in maintaining evoked histamine release.

Strontium not only will replace calcium but may also be more effective, since a greater maximum histamine release is observed in the presence of strontium than in calcium. Foreman and Mongar (1972) have concluded from kinetic analysis that calcium and strontium act on similar sites and that strontium has a greater "efficacy" at these sites. Barium, while also capable of replacing calcium, requires higher concentrations than strontium. The simi-lar affinity constants of calcium for the "calcium receptor" in mast cells and motor nerve terminals may be merely fortuitous, but it also may mean that the role of calcium in activating histamine release is similar to that in activating transmitter release. This similarity would also imply that in the mast cell calcium acts at the stage between the changes produced by the stimulating effect of the antigen–antibody reaction and the degranulation process, although it does not necessarily imply that degranulation and histamine release are processes initiated by a triggering event on the surface membrane of the mast cell.

Further insight into the ionic events associated with histamine release from mast cells has come from studies involving the releasing activity of the polymer substance 48/80 and ATP. The stimulant action of both 48/80 and ATP is dependent on calcium (Diamant and Krüger, 1967). However, histamine release induced by 48/80 seems less calcium dependent, since in some systems calcium is not an absolute requirement for the action of 48/80, although the presence of calcium enhances the release (cf. Rubin, 1970; Strandberg, 1971). The calcium dependence of the histamine releasing effect of 48/80 appears to vary with the tissue and the species. Thus histamine release from isolated rat peritoneal mast cells by 48/80 is unaffected by calcium lack. By contrast, ATP-induced histamine release from isolated mast cells of the rat depends on the presence of calcium and is inhibited by magnesium (Sugiyama, 1971). Both ATP and 48/80 require energy for releasing activity (Diamant and Uvnäs, 1961; Diamant and Peterson, 1970), as does antigen-induced release (Chakravarty, 1962); however, available data suggest that glycolytic energy production is sufficient for 48/80-induced release, whereas histamine release induced by extracellular ATP requires functioning oxidative phorylation; this may imply basic differences in the mode of action of these two agents. Moreover, any conclusions drawn concerning physiological events from the use of pharmcological agents must be considered in light of the fact that in many instances pharmacologically induced release may be occurring through entirely different mechanisms and thus may be fundamentally different from the release occurring through the normal physiological channels.

With this precaution in mind, let us see what additional evidence obtained with antigen- as well as 48/80- and ATP-induced histamine release tells us about the events associated with this specific secretory process. In systems so far considered, membrane stimulation appears to be associated with permeability changes which may be measured by electrophysiological techniques. Indeed, depolarization of the rat mesentery mast cell follows the addition of 48/80 or ATP (Tasaka *et al.*, 1970). However, the electrophysiological changes do not appear to be temporally correlated with secretory events in that degranulation can be demonstrated before depolarization, although degranulation continues after complete depolarization. These data suggest that depolarization is not a causal phenomenon in the mechanism of mast cell degranulation but—as in other secretory systems—merely a secondary event.

Direct studies of the changes in ionic distribution which occur concomitantly with histamine release are not numerous and do little to clarify the ionic events which occur during stimulation. However, the evidence adduced up to now seems to indicate that stimulation of the rat mast cell by 48/80 or ATP results in an increase in calcium and sodium uptake and an enhancement of potassium release (Dahlquist and Diamant, 1972). ATP-stimulated calcium uptake precedes histamine release, but release induced by ATP seems to be a combination of an increased entry of both sodium and calcium. The role of sodium again may be related to an effect on calcium distribution, since Unväs and his associates, while demonstrating that 48/80 also causes an increase in ^{22}Na uptake by mast cells, concluded from the time course of sodium uptake and the amount of sodium entering the mast cells that the intracellular accumulation of sodium and histamine release are not directly related (Slorach and Uvnäs, 1969). On the other hand, sodium uptake is not secondary to histamine release, since sodium uptake reaches a maximum before ATP-induced histamine release becomes apparent.

In mast cells, granule-bound histamine is stored in an ionic linkage to a heparin–protein complex (Uvnäs et al., 1970). Uvnäs has proposed that histamine release induced by 48/80 is a two-step process: an energy-requiring degranulation to the outside of the cell, followed by histamine release from granules; the latter process is thought to be a nonenzymatic ion exchange between extracellular cations and histamine in the extruded granules (Thon and Uvnäs, 1967). However, since the release of histamine from mast cells in response to 48/80 involves the extrusion of other granule constituents, including the histamine-carrying heparin–protein complex, the mast cell response resembles the processes involved in the release of other granule-bound, biologically active substances (Fillion et al., 1970). Thus Uvnäs's theory of histamine release, if valid, should also apply to the release of other biogenic amines, but most of the evidence which has accumulated indicates that following medullary catecholamine release the chromaffin granule membrane remains within the chromaffin cell (cf. Kirshner and Kirshner, 1971; Smith and Winkler, 1972).

5-Hydroxytryptamine

5-Hydroxytryptamine (5-HT) is localized in blood platelets, which play an important role in hemostasis by forming aggregates. Platelets contain two main types of granules: one involved with the storage of 5-HT and one related to a lysosome-like particle. The hormone-storing granules also contain large concentrations of adenine nucleotide (Holmsen *et al.*, 1972) and calcium (Mürer and Holme, 1970)—which are also stored with catecholamine in the chromaffin granules of the adrenal medulla—suggesting that storage mechanisms for biogenic amines are essentially similar. The adenine nucleotide (mainly ATP) and calcium are probably required for the formation of a binding complex with the amine. This is indicated by *in vitro* studies which show that mixtures of nucleotide and amine form molecular aggregates with calcium, while the amine alone does not aggregate with these metal ions (Berneis *et al.*, 1971). Thus the 5-HT-storing organelle is viewed as a structure having a high concentration of bivalent cation and nucleotide which incorporates the amine into the molecular aggregate after it is taken up into the granules.

The term "platelet release reaction" was introduced by Grette in 1962 to describe the explosive sequence of events by which platelets release their granular constituents to the surrounding medium following stimulation. Associated with the release of the cellular components, platelet aggregation is induced (Mustard and Packham, 1970). Platelet release can be induced by antigen, thrombin, or a variety of other miscellaneous substances, including trypsin, collagen, snake venom, and biogenic amines (Davey and Lüscher, 1968; Holmsen *et al.*, 1969). The mode of action of these stimulating agents is not well understood, but an effect on the cell membrane is considered most likely. Thrombin, the enzyme that catalyzes conversion of fibrinogen to fibrin, is one of the most potent stimulators of platelet releasing activity; the rapid effect of thrombin is associated with the release of 5-HT, adenine nucleotide, and calcium, but only a small amount of protein (Holmsen and Day, 1970; Mürer and Holme, 1970). The presumption that the source of the released adenine nucleotide and calcium is an intracellular granular binding site is supported by the findings that the released nucleotide is metabolically inert and that the calcium emanates from a stored form inaccessible to exchange with the extracellular medium. The general pattern of calcium release closely follows the pattern of adenine nucleotide release and affirms that calcium is stored in the same granules as 5-HT and ATP (Mürer and Holme, 1970).

The parallel release of 5-HT and nucleotide in approximately the same proportion as they exist in subcellular particles suggests that 5-HT release from platelets occurs by extrusion of material located in granules directly to the external medium. The specificity of the permeability change is supported by the finding that there is no increase in the extracellular distribution of enzymes, such as lactic dehydrogenase, which are presumed to be present in the soluble part of the platelet (Holmsen and Day, 1970). On the other hand, the release reaction is associated with the extrusion of lysosomal enzymes, which are also sequestered in granules (Davey and Lüscher, 1968).

It will become apparent that selective release from cell organelles, which is related to the discharge of components directly from membrane-limited granules within the cell interior without discharge of granules themselves, is a fairly general biological phenomenon. The similarity in the platelet release reaction with other secretory systems might indicate that this system—like others it resembles—involves a calcium-dependent process. And indeed release induced by low concentrations of thrombin is blocked by chelating agents such as EDTA. If platelets treated with thrombin in the presence of EDTA are washed and resuspended, release occurs on the addition of calcium (Sneddon, 1972; cf. Rubin, 1970). This phenomenon is analogous to the release reaction of leukocytes, which will be discussed subsequently. This latter system can be primed by exposure to leucocidin and triggered by the addition of calcium.

The mere omission of calcium from the incubation medium is not always sufficient to markedly depress 5-HT release, and even chelating agents do not completely inhibit release of platelet constituents by high concentrations of thrombin. However, the ability of high concentrations of stimulating agents to release in the absence of calcium is now a well-documented phenomenon and may indicate a releasing activity through nonphysiological mechanisms. For example, some releasing agents—especially in high concentrations—act by causing lysis of platelets, which may explain, at least in part, the lack of calcium dependency with high concentrations of stimulant. But, for whatever the reason, it is apparent that high concentrations of stimulant will under certain conditions limit the calcium requirement, even in a system which under normal physiological conditions appears to be calcium dependent.

The release of 5-HT from platelets manifests responses to alterations in the ionic milieu generally similar to those observed in other secretory organs. Thus strontium and barium can substitute for calcium in thrombin-induced release from rat blood platelets although barium is somewhat less active, while magnesium inhibits secretion (Sneddon, 1972). The removal of potassium has no effect on release, but the removal of sodium decreases calcium-dependent release by approximately 50%; however, the inhibition of thrombin-induced release under conditions of sodium deprivation is less marked when high concentrations of thrombin are employed, which again demonstrates that ionic dependencies may be bypassed during supramaximal stimulation.

There is little evidence available that would really help us to understand which changes in the pattern of ion distribution, if any, are mainly responsible for the platelet release reaction. In addition to the well-documented increase in calcium efflux, there is also an augmented magnesium efflux (Tidball and Scherer, 1972). Both of these cations are present in the secretory granule to aid in the binding of biogenic amine, so it is not surprising that they are being released along with the other constituents of the organelle. But these findings are difficult to reconcile with the report that thrombin-induced release can also be associated with a net increase in platelet calcium (Kinlough-Rathbone et al., 1973). Sodium, like calcium, appears to be required for the release reaction in rat blood platelets; but in rabbit platelets, where potassium efflux and histamine release appear to be related events, no net sodium movement is discernible, indicating that release can occur independently of net sodium transfer (Tidball et al., 1971).

It is obvious from the meager amount of data presently available that any discussion of the ionic-dependent events operating during the platelet-release reaction would be highly speculative. However, the need for calcium-chelating agents to uncover the requirement for calcium on intact platelets suggests that a store of calcium not readily exchangeable with the extracellular milieu may be involved in the release process. This possibility gains credence by the finding that platelets contain an ATP-dependent, calcium-dependent binding protein, which in some respects appears to be similar to the sarcoplasmic reticulum of skeletal muscle (Statland *et al.*, 1969). Such a system may provide the source of the calcium involved in initiating the platelet release reaction.

Not only has the specific calcium fraction involved with release not been clearly defined, but the site of calcium action is also still a matter of debate. Some insight into the role of calcium may be provided by the fact that the platelet release reaction, like so many other secretory phenomena, requires energy; this energy requirement is not just to maintain the platelet in a viable condition, but for a more specific purpose which may involve an interaction of the high-energy phosphate compound with calcium.

Grette (1962) originally suggested that the platelet release reaction—which is important for hemostasis—involves a process analogous to muscle contraction. This contractile event in platelets is mediated by thrombosthenin, a complex of proteins that shares many characteristics with muscle actin and myosin (Lüscher *et al.*, 1972). Like actomyosin from striated muscle, to which it is closely related, thrombosthenin shows Ca^{2+}- and Mg^+-dependent ATPase activity and spontaneous contraction at low ionic strength in the presence of ATP and magnesium (Bettex-Galland and Lüscher, 1965). It has been suggested that contractile ATPase stimulated by ATP may, as in muscle, give rise to contractions, resulting in the extrusion of granules (Grette, 1962). It is of interest that calcium is a very potent activator and magnesium, at high concentrations, an inhibitor of thrombosthenin ATPase (Bettex-Galland and Lüscher, 1965). Thus Grette's (1962) original idea, that calcium ATP and contractile protein may be a critical step in secretion as well as muscle contraction, has taken on added validity, and will be considered again in the next chapter.

RELEASE OF WATER AND PROTEIN

Salivary Gland

After considering many secretory systems, it is apparent that most, if not all, operate via some calcium-dependent mechanism, although the concept of stimulus–secretion coupling may not be rigidly applicable in every case. Such a situation appears to obtain in the salivary glands. These organs, which include the submaxillary, sublingual, and parotid glands, exhibit a great degree of morphological complexity and secrete both water and electrolytes as well as protein in response to parasympathetic and sympathetic nerve stimulation (Schneyer *et al.*, 1972). Amylase is one of the proteins secreted by these exocrine glands, and a majority of it is found in the zymogen granule fraction. The sequence of events which occurs in regard to salt and water secretion is complicated by the fact that along with secretion there is reabsorption in the duct systems, which is analogous to the renal reabsorptive mechanism (Schneyer *et al.*, 1972). Thus in the acinar cells a primary secretion occurs which is of a composition similar to the sodium, potassium, and chloride concentrations of plasma. In the duct system a net reabsorption of sodium chloride occurs, and also a secretion of potassium. Moreover, ion concentrations of saliva are determined by flow rates; for example, saliva may become more hypertonic with increasing flow rates as the reabsorptive capacity of the duct cells is exceeded. Therefore, the ability of the secretomotor parasympathetic fibers to produce wide changes in salivary flow rates may complicate interpretations of secretory events occurring under various experimental conditions.

Although Douglas and Poisner (1963) first demonstrated that the salivary secretion fundamentally involves a calcium-dependent process, membrane events and ion fluxes did not always parallel those which occur in medullary chromaffin cells or secretory neurons. Using the perfused cat submaxillary gland, they found that the output of water and protein, in response to acetylcholine, varied with the extracellular calcium concentration over the range of 0–8 mM, although the output of protein was more severely impaired by the omission of calcium. The effect of calcium deprivation was readily reversible, and 20 min after reintroducing calcium the secretory response to acetylcholine was restored. When the calcium concentration was increased fourfold the protein output was augmented, but the high calcium did not affect the volume or electrolyte content of the saliva evoked by acetylcholine. Although Douglas and Poisner saw similarities in the effects of calcium on salivary secretion with those of the adrenal medulla, they also realized that other observed phenomena did not make a strong case for the simple conclusion that calcium acts as a link in "stimulus–secretion coupling" in the salivary gland in a manner parallel to its action at the adrenal medulla. The idea that calcium acts by entering the acinar cells to trigger salivary secretion was weakened by the findings that the stimulant effect of reintroducing calcium following a period of calcium deprivation was not regularly seen, and the depression of salivary secretion produced by excess magnesium was very small when compared to its blockade of medullary secretion. One of the suggestions proposed by these investigators was that calcium might influence the membrane events associated with extrusion of electrolytes and proteins.

The importance of calcium for protein secretion has been affirmed on rodent parotid glands *in vitro* (Ishida *et al.*, 1971), and for salivary secretion on perfused cat submandibular glands (Petersen *et al.*, 1967), although there is another report that enzyme secretion from rat parotid slices induced by epinephrine does not require calcium in the medium (Batzri and Selinger, 1973). This latter finding suggests that the critical calcium fraction may not be localized to the extracellular fluid but may be bound in some cellular site, so that the calcium requirement may be met through the leakage of calcium from cellular stores. Such potential stores exist in the microsomal fraction, which avidly binds calcium *in vitro* (Selinger *et al.*, 1970), and in the amylase-containing secretory granules, which sequester large amounts of exportable protein (Wallach and Schramm, 1971).

Petersen has carried out kinetic studies to ascertain the localization of the critical calcium fraction, and he found that during the first few minutes of perfusing the cat submandibular gland with a calcium-free medium salivary secretion does not decrease significantly but is rapidly abolished during perfusion with low-sodium solution (Martinez and Petersen, 1972); these findings indicate that the salivary secretory rate does not depend on extracellular calcium but does depend on extracellular sodium and that acetylcholine-induced calcium influx is not the triggering mechanism for the initiation of the secretory process. The rapid diminution in the salivary secretory response after sodium deprivation indicates that, unlike the secretory systems previously discussed, sodium apparently plays a more direct and immediate role.

Electrophysiological studies have also provided us with insight into the nature of the ionic events. The resting membrane potential of the salivary gland is approximately −20 mV (Schneyer *et al.*, 1972), and the addition of acetylcholine generally results in a hyperpolarization up to −50 mV; this hyperpolarization (called the secretory potential) is not always observed, but at times depolarization is the major potential change. The hyperpolarization could be due to a net increase in anion influx into the acinar cell or to a net increase in cation efflux. Lundberg (1958) originally showed that the salivary secretory rate was dependent on the chloride concentration of the perfusion fluid, and he postulated that an active transport of chloride ions into the cell is the primary step in salivary secretion. However, this concept is mitigated by the finding that the replacement of chloride with the impermeant anion, sulfate, diminishes secretion, but the secretory potential remains intact (Petersen, 1971).

Much more evidence has accumulated to support the idea that potassium efflux is a critical ionic event associated with salivary secretion. Burgen (1956) first described the loss of potassium into the saliva as a prominent feature of the early phase of evoked salivary secretion, and Schneyer (1967) found that cholinergic stimulation increased the uptake and release of radioactive potassium (^{42}K) from salivary glands, which indicates an increase in potassium conductance. Although the slope of the change in resting membrane potential in relation to the logarithm of the potassium concentration is appreciably less than the 60 mV predicted from the Nernst equation for a potassium electrode, elevation of extracellular potassium abolishes the secretory potentials (Petersen, 1971) and inhibits secretion by diminishing the electrochemical gradient for potassium (Petersen and Poulsen, 1967). Thus the present view of membrane activation of the salivary acinar cell, for which Petersen has been such a strong proponent, is that the initial effect of acetylcholine on the acinar cell is to cause an increase in potassium permeability (Petersen, 1971); this effect of cholinergic stimulation on potassium permeability in salivary glands parallels its action on the heart, where the negative inotropic action of vagal stimulation is also mediated through an increase in potassium permeability (Trautwein and Dudel, 1958). Sodium fluxes are also enhanced by the action of acetylcholine and result in the short-circuiting of the potassium current, as evidenced by the finding that the size of the secretory potential increases when the extracellular sodium is replaced by the impermeant cation, tetraethylammonium (Petersen, 1971). Thus the acinar cells appear to be quite different from chromaffin cells and neurons in that the sodium current does not provide the major source of cation for carrying the ionic current during membrane activation.

The significance of the inhibitory secretory potentials in controlling the secretory process is still a matter of debate; however, they can be dissociated from salivary secretion. The potential itself—but not secretion—remains after calcium deprivation when sulfate is substituted for chloride, or when the metabolic inhibitor, dinitrophenol, is added (Petersen et al., 1967; Petersen, 1971). The latter finding indicates that acinar membrane stimulation is associated with a decrease in membrane resistance and a passive flow of ions. However, despite the fact that dissociation of the electrical events from the secretory process is possible, the difficulty in dissociating these two events indicates that they are closely coupled. Thus an increase in external potassium decreases the hyperpolarizing effect of acetylcholine by reducing the electrochemical gradient. This might decrease the salivary secretory rate by diminishing sodium influx, which appears to be a critical event leading to salivary secretion (cf. Petersen, 1970, 1971).

Although it is apparent that ionic events other than those involving calcium must also be considered as crucial to the extrusion process, one cannot overlook the fact that in the absence of calcium salivary glands are unable to secrete. Moreover, parasympathetic stimulants enhance radiocalcium uptake and efflux in a variety of salivary gland preparations (Dreisbach, 1964; Nielsen and Petersen, 1972). However, the role of this calcium transport in the secretory response is obscure since the calcium uptake is magnesium dependent, although magnesium depresses the secretory response to acetylcholine (Nielsen and Petersen,

1972). The acetylcholine-induced increase in calcium efflux is observed under conditions where the gland is unable to secrete, e.g., after calcium-free or sodium-free perfusion. These findings suggest that acetylcholine action results in the release of bound calcium from cellular sites, with the resultant export of calcium to the external fluid.

Thus the nature of the ionic events occurring in the salivary gland appears much more complicated than that taking place in the adrenal chromaffin cell or cholinergic neurons. It is apparent from the varied findings that it has not been established whether the critical calcium fraction resides in the extra- or intracellular environment. Moreover, separate activator mechanisms may exist for fluid secretion and protein secretion. Sodium entry may increase salt and water transport, whereas calcium release may stimulate protein secretion. Such a notion is consistent with the findings of Case and Clausen (1971) in the exocrine pancreas, where acetylcholine—which increases protein secretion—increases radiocalcium release, whereas secretin— which stimulates mainly ion and water transport—exerts no effect on calcium release. Thus the difficulty in interpreting the data rests not only with the diversity of the cell types and the relative role of calcium metabolism in each cell type—which is a constant problem in all tissues—but also these complexities are multiplied in the salivary gland by the fact that there are two diverse secretory processes triggered by the same physiological stimulus.

However, the temporal dispersion of the effects of calcium deprivation on fluid and protein secretion certainly points to the fact the nature of calcium's action in their release is probably not the same. A clue to the action of calcium may lie in the existence of the powerful calcium-accumulating mechanism in the microsomal fraction (Selinger et al., 1970). This may be the source of the calcium released during acetylcholine stimulation and may explain the slow decline in the secretory response after the onset of calcium deprivation. The increase in cellular sodium produced by the chemical transmitter may augment free calcium in the cytosol by increasing calcium influx or slowing calcium efflux through sodium–calcium exchange. The increase in free cell calcium may activate the sodium pump leading to sodium release, with water following passively.

On the other hand, the importance of calcium in secretion of water may be merely to retain the normal permeability conditions of the acinar cell by affecting intercellular junctions or cell membrane permeability. Many membranes require calcium for the active or passive movement of monovalent ions and for associated water movement. Thus the passive entry of sodium into the axon during the action potential is largely inactivated in the absence of calcium (Frankenhaeuser and Hodgkin, 1957), and active transport of sodium in frog skin (Curran and Gill, 1962) and rat intestine requires calcium (Dumont et al., 1960). By contrast, protein secretion appears to occur by means of exocytosis, and calcium may exert its effects on this process by facilitating the interaction of the secretory granule membrane with the cell membrane. This latter concept will be more fully discussed in Chapter 3.

Exocrine Pancreas

The pancreas, like the salivary gland, also performs an exocrine function. It contains acinar and duct cells which secrete water and electrolytes, as well as digestive enzymes, into the small intestine. The protein is contained within the zymogen granules, and their role in the secretory process has been elucidated by the elegant studies of Palade and his associates (Palade, 1959; Jamieson and Palade, 1967). Secretory product is apparently synthesized within the cisternae of the rough endoplasmic reticulum and is then transported to the Golgi region, where it is incorporated into the immature zymogen granule. The granules then mature into secretory granules and eventually discharge their contents to the cell exterior by exocytosis.

Although there are some variations from species to species, it is generally agreed that vagal stimulation (or acetylcholine) and pancreozymin increase protein release, whereas secretin enhances mainly water and electrolyte release. Although acetylcholine is presumed to be the chemical transmitter substance responsible for protein secretion by the pancreas, it has not been identified in the effluent after vagal stimulation.

The role of calcium in the secretion of protein from the salivary gland has already been discussed, so that a complete recapitulation of the requirement for calcium in pancreatic amylase secretion would be redundant. It is sufficient to say that the original finding by Hokin (1966), that acetylcholine-induced secretion of amylase from pigeon pancreas is calcium dependent, has been corroborated in other pancreatic preparations (Benz *et al.*, 1972; Kanno, 1972), with Kanno (1972) establishing a linear relationship between the reciprocal of pancreozymin-induced amylase release and the reciprocal of the calcium concentration, with half-maximal amylase release obtained with 5 m*M* calcium (Fig. 11). Additional consideration of this system is indicated by the very interesting finding of Argent *et al.* (1971) that excess potassium stimulates amylase secretion from the perfused cat pancreas; however, unlike its action on the adrenal medulla, the stimulatory action is not due to a direct effect on the acinar cell but rather to the release of acetylcholine from the vagal nerve endings, as evidenced by the fact that its secretory activity is blocked by the cholinergic antagonist, atropine.

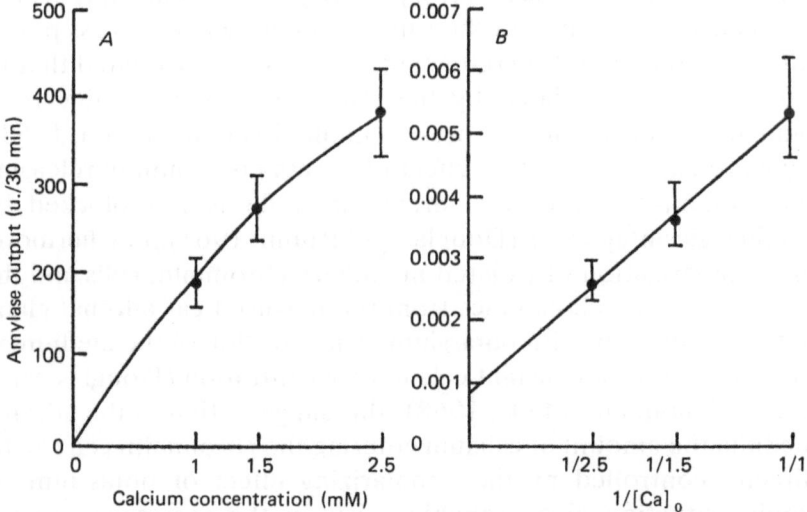

Fig. 11. Relation between amylase release evoked by pancreozymin and the calcium concentration of the medium perfusing the rat pancreas *in vitro*. B depicts Lineweaver–Burk plot for the relation shown in A (Kanno, 1972).

This finding is not so remarkable if one relates it to the early work of Brown and Feldberg (1936), who showed that excess potassium is able to enhance acetylcholine release from nerve endings, presumably by locally depolarizing them. However, what is more significant is that excess potassium, though not capable of evoking secretion through a direct action, is able to directly depolarize the acinar cell (Petersen and Matthews, 1972). This implies that depolarization is not a sufficient stimulus for acinar cell secretion. Yet the physiological stimulants acetylcholine and pancreozymin, also depolarize the acinar cell membrane (Matthews and Petersen, 1973), suggesting that an underlying permeability change may be the first step in the sequence of events leading to protein release. Thus here we have another secretory system that sustains the concept that in secretory cells depolarization is an *effect* rather than a *cause* of the increase in cation permeability which results from cell stimulation.

The finding that the stimulant effect of excess potassium on the pancreatic acinar cell is indirect has another important implication, for it raises the possibility that in other systems regulated by neuronal influences the secretory activity of potassium may also be indirect. For example, in the salivary gland, where excess potassium is also a potent secretogogue, it has been postulated that its effect may be mediated by the release of catecholamine from sympathetic nerve endings present in the tissue (Schramm, 1968). By contrast, the stimulant effect of excess potassium in releasing catecholamines from the adrenal medulla is not blocked by cholinergic antagonists (Douglas and Rubin, 1961). Furthermore, the depolarization of isolated medullary chromaffin cells and the secretion of catecholamines from the perfused cat adrenal gland both vary directly with potassium concentration of the medium in the presence of a constant calcium concentration (Douglas *et al.*, 1967b; Rubin and Miele, 1968); this suggests that in the adrenal medulla the amount of calcium entering the chromaffin cell can be directly controlled by the depolarizing effect of potassium. A similar situation also probably exists in the secretory neuron, where within a certain concentration range there is a linear relationship between the potassium concentration and acetylcholine release, as measured by an increase in the frequency of the miniature end-plate potential (Liley, 1956) (Fig. 5).

Such findings have raised the question of whether secretory tissues of neural origin might all be directly stimulated by potassium, whereas other secretory tissues are not. However, evidence from the endocrine pancreas tends to weaken this idea; for the reported effects of potassium on insulin secretion are not mediated via the parasympathetic nerves which innervate the islet cells, since atropine has no effect on insulin secretion stimulated by high concentrations of potassium (Hales and Milner, 1968a). But whether or not potassium acts directly on nonneurogenic secretory cells, it may be that the stimulant effect of potassium does not reside solely in its depolarizing action, because even in the cholinergic nerve ending the progressive increase in miniature end-plate potential frequency continues to develop even after maximal depolarization is attained (Gage and Quastel, 1965). This proposed second action of potassium may be a consequence of an effect on synthesis or mobilization of secretory product.

Granular Proteins from Leukocytes

In considering the effects of calcium on protein secretion, one must not overlook another protein-secreting system, the polymorphonuclear leukocyte, where investigations have raised another important issue. Here it is not yet resolved whether calcium acts at the surface of the cell membrane or must penetrate into the cell to produce its effects on the secretory process. The calcium dependence of protein secretion from rabbit and human leukocytes has been comprehensively studied by Woodin and Wieneke (Woodin, 1968), and on the basis of their investigations they have developed a model to distinguish between these two possibilities, so that their studies warrant additional consideration.

Staphylococcal leucocidin is thought to trigger secretion of lysosomal protein by inducing changes in the leukocyte that mimic those in excitable or secretory tissues. In this system the excitation events appear to be clearly separated from the secretory events, for if leucocidin is added in the absence of calcium the stimulating events are initiated, as evidenced by the fact that secretion can be subsequently induced by the addition of calcium following neutralization of leucocidin with antibody. The stimulatory events associated with leucocidin stimulation have not been clearly elaborated, although they are thought to somehow involve transport of potassium (Woodin and Wieneke, 1968).

The secretory events which occur in the presence of calcium include secretion of granule protein consisting of β-glucosidase, ribonuclease, and peroxidase, an accumulation of calcium within the cell, and a splitting of organic phosphate (Woodin and Wieneke, 1963). If leucocidin-treated cells are maintained in a calcium-deprived state, secretion of granule enzymes does not occur, but the cell becomes permeable to cytoplasmic enzymes such as aldolase. The efficiency of calcium as the inducer of protein secretion decreases as the time of incubating the leucocidin-treated cells in a calcium-free medium is increased (Woodin and Wieneke, 1963). However, the secretory activity can be augmented by the addition of nucleotides to the calcium-deprived medium. This indicates a critical relationship between calcium and ATP in the events associated with protein release.

Another interesting conclusion drawn by these investigators is that the calcium which accumulates in the cell after stimulation is not a consequence of calcium penetration into the cytoplasm through an increase in cell membrane permeability (Woodin and Wieneke, 1970). Calcium is perceived to occupy specific sites on the inside of the cell membrane to facilitate interaction of the membrane of the secretory granule with cell membrane, which culminates in the release of protein by exocytosis. According to this scheme, once adherence of the membrane has occurred, calcium must be removed from site of contact, and this is accomplished by its combining with the orthophosphate formed from splitting of ATP. The calcium–phosphate complex is then presumed to be taken up by the vesicles.

This concept of protein secretion has been presented, even though the evidence supporting it is far from conclusive, because it represents another plausible way of envisaging the calcium-dependent events which lead to the extrusion of secretory product. In this view, the effect of the stimulating agent is associated with a translocation of calcium to specific membrane sites rather than a general transmembrane flux.

Even if the tenuous conclusions of Woodin and Wieneke are valid for protein secretion from the leukocyte, it still raises the question as to whether this model can be extended to other secretory systems. Mitochondria and endoplasmic reticulum are less prominent in the leukocyte than in many other secretory cells. Since these organelles are generally utilized to sequester calcium, this lack may necessitate that the leukocyte develop an alternative mechanism for effecting secretion. The finding that the optimal calcium concentration (0.1 mM) for protein secretion is lower than that observed in most other secretory systems would be consistent with an inadequate system to maintain cell calcium at low levels (Woodin and Wieneke, 1963). On the other hand, the ability of magnesium to inhibit leucocidin-induced protein secretion indicates that protein secretion from leukocytes apparently has certain basic characteristics in common with the secretory process in other tissues (Woodin and Wienke, 1964). Obviously, additional experimentation is required to determine whether calcium acts at the level of the cell membrane or at some intracellular site, but both possibilities should be considered as viable alternatives.

GASTRIC SECRETION

Although there is no doubt that calcium exerts a direct and definitive action on the machinery which activates the secretory apparatus, it is also apparent from the foregoing discussion that its effects on other parameters of cell function which indirectly affect normal secretory activity may at times make it difficult to dissociate any indirect effects from its more direct action on the secretory process. Therefore, a blockade of secretion following a period of calcium deprivation is not *prima facie* evidence that calcium is directly involved in the release process, even if the block can be readily reversed by the readdition of calcium. This point is best illustrated by considering the effects of calcium on gastric secretion.

In 1941 Gray and Adkinson, on the basis of calcium deprivation studies, suggested that calcium somehow affected the secretory process and electrical parameters of the frog gastric mucosa. Forte and Nauss (1963) later found that exposure to calcium-free solutions bathing the nutrient and secretory sides of the frog gastric mucosa leads to a decrease in the transmembrane potential, in the membrane resistance, and in the rate of acid secretion. These investigators did not explain the effects of calcium as a result of a direct effect on the gastric secretory mechanism but rather as being due to calcium depletion affecting the intercellular binding between cells. They reasoned that the effect of calcium deprivation was akin to that observed in frog skin, where calcium deprivation enhances passive ion permeability through the skin by an increased permeability in the intercellular spaces. Jacobson *et al.* (1965) repeated the experiments of Forte and Nauss, and were able to demonstrate two phases of secretory failure during calcium deprivation. The removal of calcium from solutions bathing the isolated frog gastric mucosa resulted in an initial increase in resistance accompanied by a 50% fall in acid secretion after transmural stimulation. These effects were followed by a second phase which was characterized by a pronounced decrease in resistance and a fall in acid secretion to zero. A complete reversal of the second phase was obtained on the readdition of calcium.

Jacobson and his colleagues advanced the most plausible explanation for these findings by suggesting that permeability is not radically altered during the initial stage of calcium deprivation, as evidenced by the increase in membrane resistance, and that during the first phase the removal of calcium reduces the rate of acid secretion by a direct effect on the secretory mechanism. The decrease in resistance during the second phase may be the result of an increase in permeability due to a widening of the intercellular spaces when calcium is removed from the bathing solution.

If calcium is directly involved with gastric secretion, then the secretory rate should bear some relationship to the calcium concentration. Such quantitative studies are lacking in *in vitro* studies, although the ability of calcium administration to augment gastric secretion in man is a well-known clinical finding and probably accounts for the high incidence of peptic ulcers in the syndrome of hyperparathyroidism, which is associated with hypercalcemia. The administration of calcium not only produces an increase in acid output but also augments pepsin and gastrin secretion (Barreras and Donaldson, 1967; Trudeau and McGuigan, 1969).

Since acid secretion is regulated by both neural and hormonal influences, such studies *in vivo* do little to elucidate the site of calcium action. The ability of hypermagnesemia to block the effects of hypercalcemia on gastric secretion (Barreras and Donaldson, 1967) suggests that one is dealing with a secretory mechanism which is similar, at least in certain respects, to those observed in most other systems. However, the hypercalcemic effect on gastric secretion can be blocked by surgical denervation or by pharmacological denervation with the use of atropine (Smallwood, 1967), which may indicate that the calcium effects are mediated through acetylcholine release from the vagus nerve. Another question still left unanswered is whether the actions of calcium on acid secretion are mediated through a direct effect on the acid-producing parietal cells or are mediated indirectly through the release of gastrin, which in turn stimulates the parietal cell.

These are very important questions to be answered, since the secretory process in the parietal cell may be quite different from that of the protein-secreting gastric zymogen cells. The latter are very similar to the pancreatic acinar cells, from both a morphological and a functional point of view, since they both contain readily visible protein-containing secretory granules which release their contents to the cell exterior by exocytosis. By contrast, the most striking characteristic of the parietal cell is the intracellular canaliculi, which open onto the apical cell surface (Helander, 1967). These structures, which have not been observed in any other normal mammalian cell, have also been demonstrated in the acid-secreting frog oxyntic cell (Forte *et al.*, 1972). Secretory product may be produced or accumulated within vacuoles which are present in great numbers in the cytoplasm of the resting parietal cell and they decrease in number after stimulation (Helander *et al.*, 1972). However, no cytological methods are yet available to ascertain whether these vacuoles do indeed contain secretory product. Another distinguishing characteristic of the morphological changes associated with acid secretion is the great increase in number of microvilli which project from the apical cell surface and may provide the means whereby substances leave the cell (Helander, 1967).

Thus any potential effect of calcium on this seemingly unusual secretory process may help us to eventually elucidate the intimate role of this cation in triggering the events leading to secretion. On the other hand, if the vacuoles do contain secretory product, they may migrate to the plasma membrane, where they empty their contents into the lumen in a manner analogous to that observed during exocytosis, so that one may not have to explain the mechanism of calcium action on the basis of diverse mechanisms of secretion. A final possibility, which will be discussed in further detail in the next chapter, involves the tubular components of the cell as a potential site of calcium action.

ENDOCRINE SECRETORY SYSTEMS

The Douglas (1968) concept of stimulus–secretion coupling states that glands are caused to secrete by the entry of calcium into the cell, which is brought about by changes in the permeability properties of the plasma membrane. The adrenal medulla has been considered the prototype of glands which utilize such a mechanism. The medullary chromaffin cells are somewhat unique in that they are of neurological ancestry, but, unlike neurosecretory and more conventional neurons, they respond to chemical rather than electrical stimulation; yet they resemble neurons by responding to challenges with depolarizing concentrations of potassium, as long as calcium is present in the medium. The action of the chemical transmitter agent, acetylcholine, on the chromaffin cell is also associated with depolarization, although calcium entry rather than depolarization *per se* appears to be the critical event. In light of the relation of chromaffin cells to neuronal tissue, the question arises as to whether secretogogues of nonneurogenic endocrine glands also act through a mechanism which is consistent with the concept of stimulus–secretion coupling.

Insulin Release

The endocrine function of the pancreas involves the regulation of metabolic activity through the actions of insulin and glucagon, which are synthesized, stored, and released from the

β and α cells, respectively. The importance of calcium for insulin secretion is well documented from studies *in vitro* with isolated perfused rat pancreas (Curry *et al.*, 1968a), pieces of rabbit pancreas (Hales, 1971), and organ cultures of fetal rat pancreas (Lambert *et al.*, 1969a). A variety of chemically dissimilar compounds in addition to the physiological stimulus, glucose, are able to augment insulin release; these agents include the oral hypoglycemic agents such as tolbutamide, amino acids (such as leucine), potassium, and ouabain (Grodsky, 1970); the stimulant actions of all of the above agents are reversibly inhibited by the absence of calcium (Randle and Hales, 1972).

Curry *et al.* (1968b) employed the perfused rat pancreas to study the effects of calcium on the dynamics of insulin secretion by measuring changes in the rate of insulin released during constant stimulation (Fig. 12). On exposure to glucose, the onset of insulin

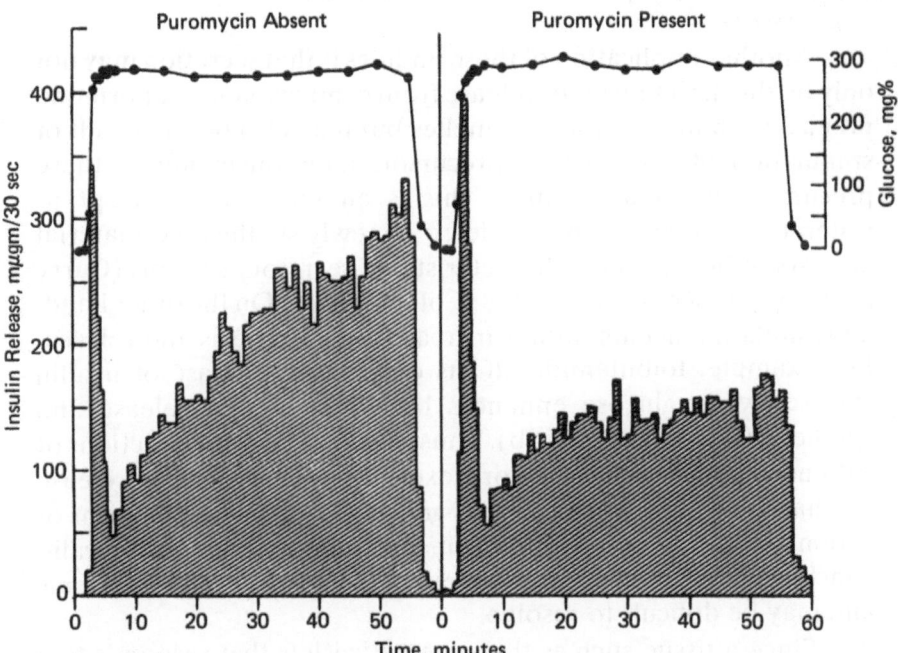

Fig. 12. Time course of insulin release from the isolated perfused rat pancreas in response to a continuous infusion of glucose, in the absence and presence of puromycin (Curry *et al.*, 1968b).

release is rapid, occurring within less than 1 min; secretion rates then decline within 5 min. This phase of insulin release is thought to be the result of release of preformed insulin, since it is not blocked by inhibitors of protein synthesis such as puromycin. After 10 min, a second, more prolonged phase of insulin release is observed which is partially blocked by puromycin, indicating that this phase is associated with insulinogenesis (Fig. 12). Both phases of insulin secretion are calcium dependent, and calcium, unlike puromycin, has no effect on the incorporation of radioactive amino acids into pancreatic protein, indicating that while calcium is required for insulin secretion, it plays no critical role in the biosynthesis of hormone. These data on the islet cells indicating that calcium has no marked effects on hormone synthesis cannot be arbitrarily transferred to certain other systems. For example, in the adrenal cortex, steroid synthesis—as well as release—depends profoundly on the presence of calcium (Jaanus *et al.*, 1970; Rubin *et al.*, 1972).

Another implication of these findings is that secretion may not only be the direct result of release from compartments of hormone prepackaged in secretory organelles but may also be the result of stimulation of synthesis of precursors and conversion of these precursors to final product. This is an important concept to reiterate, since preferential release of newly synthesized material appears to be a general characteristic of secretory systems (Curry *et al.*, 1968b; Kopin *et al.*, 1968; Collier, 1969). On the other hand, all stimulating agents do not increase both synthesis and release. For example, tolbutamide affects only the first phase of insulin release, while glucose enhances both phases, i.e., release and synthesis (Curry *et al.*, 1968b). Thus when evaluating the actions of cations—or any other factors exerting effects on the release mechanism—one should have a good idea of the mechanism of action of the given secretogogue in order to draw more valid conclusions. This complication exists in most secretory systems and may be difficult to resolve.

Since a tissue such as the pancreatic islets that responds to a variety of diverse chemicals may be activated by more than one mechanism, it would seem more profitable to consider the mode of action of glucose, the physiological secretogogue. The basic question still unresolved is whether glucose acts at the membrane level or whether it enters the β cell and provides the signal for insulin release through some metabolite. The latter concept gains support from the findings that glucose freely permeates the islet cell and the metabolizable sugars, such as mannose, stimulate insulin release, while the nonmetabolizable galactose does not (Grodsky, 1970). Inhibition of metabolism by anoxia, for example, also decreases glucose-induced insulin secretion (Grodsky, 1970), although this effect may not be the result of the inhibition of glucose metabolism but may be the result of interfering with the metabolic requirements of the release process *per se*.

Rather than viewing glucose-induced insulin release strictly in biochemical terms, others have drawn attention to the action of glucose to produce changes in the distribution of ions within various extra- and intracellular compartments of the β cell. The effects of ions in the β cell are strikingly similar to those observed in certain secretory systems where it has been conclusively shown that stimulus recognition is associated with calcium-dependent events. Thus not only is calcium required for insulin secretion, but also the amount of insulin release in response to glucose is directly related to the calcium concentration of the medium up to 2–3 mM; with higher calcium concentration the response remains constant, and above 10 mM it may be diminished (Hales and Milner, 1968b). Just as in other secretory organs, the effects of magnesium and barium have also been studied. Magnesium cannot substitute for calcium and, furthermore, inhibits secretion when added to the medium containing calcium (Hales and Milner, 1968b; Bennett *et al.*, 1969). The actions of barium on insulin secretion are in some ways similar to its effects on medullary catecholamine release. Thus barium stimulates insulin secretion, and this stimulant activity is inhibited by either calcium or magnesium (Hales and Milner, 1968b).

Such data suggest that glucose-induced insulin secretion is triggered by the influx of calcium into the β cell. In support of this concept, glucose was reported to increase the uptake of radiocalcium by isolated islets (Malaisse, 1972); moreover, this glucose-induced calcium uptake is inhibited by local anesthetics, which suppress the stimulant action of glucose on insulin release (Bressler and Brendel, 1971). Thus there exists an apparent correlation between calcium entry and insulin secretion.

If glucose stimulation is associated with changes in transmembrane cation flux, then one might expect that the resulting permeability changes produced by glucose would be represented by electrophysiological events. And indeed Dean and Matthews (1970a), using microelectrode techniques, have been able to measure changes in membrane potential of islet cells exposed to glucose. The islet cell membranes have a resting potential of about -20 mV. The addition of glucose (or tolbutamide) (Dean and Matthews, 1968) produces rapid fluctuations in the potential which resemble many features of the action potential observed in excitable cells. Analysis of these potentials indicates that although some external sodium is required for genesis of this electrical activity, the action potentials cannot be accounted for simply on the basis of sodium influx, but must also include calcium influx (Dean and Matthews, 1970b). Thus calcium depletion prevents the appearance of electrical activity, and increasing calcium increases the amplitude of the potentials. Moreover, manganese, which inhibits calcium entry in other tissues, blocks this glucose-induced electrical activity.

On the basis of such evidence, Dean and Matthews have attempted to establish a positive correlation between the ability of glucose to initiate action potential discharge in islet cells and the ability to trigger secretion (Dean and Matthews, 1970a). This does not mean that these two events are undissociably linked, as evidenced by the finding that electrical activity can be uncoupled from insulin secretion by excess magnesium—which blocks secretion but has no effect on the action potential discharge (Dean and Matthews, 1970b). This also implies that magnesium can inhibit calcium-dependent processes by an intracellular action.

Despite the findings of Dean and Matthews, caution must still be employed in ascribing importance to electrical events in secretory organs, for we have already seen that although membrane activation is associated with electrical changes, the secretory process can proceed independently of the membrane potential. So, with apologies to the electrophysiologist, I would like at this juncture to restate the postulate that the principal response of a secretory organ to stimulation involves a redistribution of ions, and the associated electrical events are only a consequence of, not a requirement for, triggering the extrusion of secretory product.

Although calcium plays a crucial and indispensable role in glucose-induced insulin release from the β-cell, just as in other secretory systems sodium plays a secondary but not insignificant role. It was Hales and Milner who provided evidence that the transport of calcium across the β-cell membrane somehow involves sodium (Hales and Milner, 1968a). They found that ouabain and potassium deprivation, which inhibit the active transport of sodium and cause an intracellular accumulation of sodium, stimulate insulin secretion. Moreover, the augmentation of secretion by these agents, as well as by glucose and tolbutamide, is inhibited by sodium deprivation. Barium also appears to be a pancreatic secretogogue only in the presence of extracellular sodium (Hales and Milner, 1968b). This finding is in marked contrast to that on the adrenal medulla, where in the absence of sodium, barium continues to act as a powerful secretogogue and can still depolarize isolated chromaffin cells (Douglas and Rubin, 1964b; Douglas *et al.*, 1967b).

On the other hand, extracellular sodium is neither a sufficient nor a necessary condition for insulin release to occur. In fact, during the first 30 min of sodium deprivation the basal release of insulin is enhanced (Hales and Milner, 1968b). Furthermore, whereas glucose is unable to stimulate insulin secretion in a calcium-free medium, it will stimulate insulin secretion in a sodium-free medium (Malaisse, 1972), and indeed glucose-induced insulin release is initially potentiated when sodium is replaced by potassium or choline (Malaisse *et al.*, 1971a). It is only when pieces of pancreas are incubated for 1 hr or more in a sodium-free medium that secretogogues become relatively ineffective. Finally, tetrodotoxin does not block insulin release stimulated by glucose, which would tend to curtail the importance of extracellular sodium (Milner and Hales, 1969), although resistance to tetrodotoxin is not by itself sufficient basis for excluding extracellular sodium as an important factor in insulin release.

The picture which thus emerges is that extracellular sodium is not essential for stimulation of insulin release, but the presence of cellular sodium does favor insulin release, and does so through effects on calcium distribution. Malaisse and his coworkers have proposed that calcium uptake is increased when sodium influx is facilitated through a ouabain-insensitive calcium–sodium exchange (Malaisse *et al.*, 1971a). The enhanced release observed during the early phase of sodium deprivation may be ascribed to the sodium–calcium competition for transport sites for entry into the β cell.

If one accepts the premise that the critical response of the β cell to glucose is an influx of extracellular calcium, then a clearer view of the events preceding the extrusion of secretory product is obtained. Yet, although Malaisse and his associates have made a strong case for the relationship between calcium uptake and insulin secretion, Hellman *et al.*, 1971, employing a different preparation and a different experimental design for determining radioactivity, have concluded that the major effect of glucose on calcium distribution—and the one which correlates better with insulin release—is to increase the amount of calcium retained in the β cell. They suggest that the site of glucose action may not be at the level of the cell membrane, but on a small fraction of the cell calcium; stimulation is presumed to cause a reallocation of this fraction to a less mobile compartment of the cell. This diversity of opinion emphasizes once again that caution must be employed in drawing conclusions from radioactive experiments which attempt to localize the redistribution of calcium—or any other ion, for that matter—to specific cell fractions.

Another possibility which cannot be ignored is that the action of glucose is associated with calcium (and sodium) entry from the extracellular fluid and that this ion influx *indirectly* activates the secretory process by releasing cell calcium. Such a conclusion is consistent with the available data and would explain the inhibitory effects of local anesthetics by a blockade of a calcium current not directly involved with triggering release but involved with releasing a pool of cell calcium. In this situation, an increase in cell sodium would also enhance release by competing with calcium for cellular binding sites in a cation exchange reaction. This concept is not without precedent, since the possibility has been considered that during activation of the contractile process the entry of extracellular calcium leads to contraction by releasing or replenishing a cellular fraction of calcium (Chapman and Niedergerke, 1970). In any event, the divergent views indicate that further experimentation is required to define more precisely the calcium pools directly involved in triggering insulin release.

Although the general discussion concerning the intimate role of calcium in the secretory process will be reserved for a later chapter, it might be more convenient at this time to indicate that biochemical analysis has demonstrated that the action of cellular calcium to regulate glucose-induced insulin secretion is not due to an alteration of glucose metabolism within the β cell (Ashcroft *et al.*, 1970), despite reports of a regulatory action of calcium on carbohydrate metabolism in several other tissues (Rasmussen and Nagata, 1970). The site of calcium action may be on the so-called microfilamentous–microtubular system, which is thought to possess contractile properties triggered by calcium (Malaisse, 1972). This system would facilitate the release of the insulin-containing granules via exocytosis. Whether this postulate is valid remains to be determined.

Corticosteroids

The stimulant action of pituitary adrenocorticotropin (ACTH) on corticosteroid production and release has been extensively investigated by studies on adrenocortical tissue *in vivo* and *in vitro*. However, the intimate mechanism by which steroid is extruded from cortical cells is poorly understood. In most secretory organs the secretory products are stored in granules or vesicles, and the release of secretory product is thought to occur by exocytosis. However, in the adrenal cortex, electron microscopic studies have so far failed to provide evidence for the existence of intracellular organelles that might act as a vehicle for the storage or extrusion of corticosteroids (Fawcett *et al.*, 1969). During stimulation of the cortex by ACTH, steroids are synthesized *de novo* and then diffuse out to the cell exterior, so that perhaps newly synthesized hormone is exported by circumventing the storage process. If ACTH-induced corticoid release is a calcium-dependent process and involves alterations in ionic fluxes across the plasma membrane, this might imply that the action of calcium is not confined to the process of exocytosis but is involved in some step fundamental to all processes.

A relationship between calcium and corticosteroid production and release was established by the early studies of Birmingham *et al.*, (1960), who demonstrated that calcium is needed for optimal steroid production and release *in vitro*. It was later suggested from studies on broken cell preparations, which did not respond to ACTH, that the action of calcium is to promote the intramitochondrial synthesis of steroid (Peron and McCarthy, 1968). However, experiments carried out on the isolated cat adrenal gland perfused *in situ* (Jaanus *et al.*, 1970; Rubin *et al.*, 1972) have shown that the effects of calcium on corticosteroid release are complicated by the fact that synthesis and release are tightly coupled; so that despite the fact that perfusion with calcium-free media obtunds both ACTH-induced synthesis and release, it is not clear whether this represents a primary effect of calcium on steroid biosynthesis or a secondary effect as the result of a primary action on the release mechanism.

The action of ACTH on the adrenal cortex represents a marked contrast to the action of acetylcholine on the adrenal medulla, where, in the cat adrenal perfused with Locke's solution, only the release process is activated by stimulation and is associated with transmembrane ion fluxes (Douglas, 1968). However, the adrenal cortical cells resemble the chromaffin cells in that excess potassium and ACTH can produce depolarization—even action potentials—of cortical tissue (Matthews and Saffran, 1968), although there is no correlation between the steroidogenic effect and the ability to cause cell depolarization (Matthews and Saffran, 1967). Thus depolarizing potassium concentrations produce no discernible increase in steroid release, and the action of ACTH is unaffected by maximum depolarizing concentrations of potassium (Jaanus *et al.*, 1970) (Fig. 13). This suggests that ACTH does not initiate steroid release by altering the permeability characteristics of the plasma membrane resulting in membrane depolarization. Yet radiocalcium studies demonstrate the ACTH action is associated with a slowing of calcium efflux (Jaanus and Rubin, 1971) (Fig. 1b), which one may interpret as a redistribution of cell calcium from a more rapidly exchanging cell

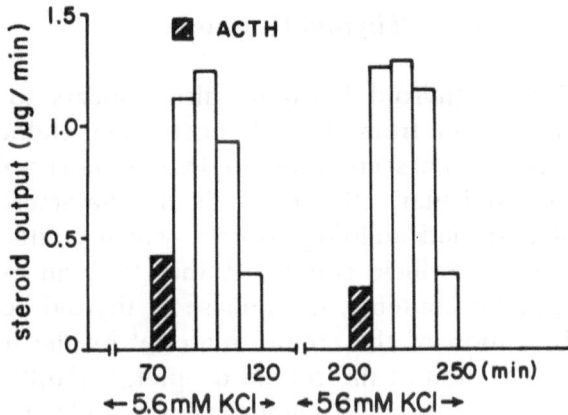

Fig. 13. The lack of effect of excess potassium on corticosteroid release from the perfused cat adrenal gland induced by ACTH (2 μU/ml) (striped bars) (Jaanus *et al.*, 1970).

fraction to one that is less readily exchangeable. Measurements of total cell calcium show no net gain in cell calcium. A slowing of calcium efflux, with no net change in total calcium, is most simply interpreted in terms of a redistribution of cell calcium.

The idea that the effects of ACTH are mediated through movements of cell calcium, rather than transmembrane ion flux, is consistent with the finding that steroid output varies with the extracellular calcium concentration up to only 0.5 mM (Jaanus *et al.*, 1970), whereas in the adrenal medulla, evoked catecholamine release is still increasing with a calcium concentration of 17.6 mM (Douglas and Rubin, 1961). Furthermore, although the secretory process of the cortex resembles that of the medulla in that strontium can replace calcium in maintaining evoked secretion, it differs qualitatively from the medulla in that barium cannot replace calcium and quantitatively in that the inhibitory effects of magnesium are less striking in the cortex (Jaanus *et al.*, 1970). Thus it appears that calcium plays some role in the release of corticosteroids, but this role may not be consistent with the stimulus–secretion coupling model proposed for the release of preformed catecholamine from the adrenal medulla.

Thyroid Hormone

Secretion of thyroid hormone also appears to involve a different mechanism from that of most other endocrine cells. Although conventional secretory granules have not been identified in the thyroid follicular cell, these cells are characterized by the presence of so-called colloid droplets, which contain material identical with the follicle colloid. Rather than an extrusion of secretory granular contents, the release of thyroid hormone involves reabsorption of the colloid material by the follicle cell, intracellular digestion of the colloid droplet, and diffusion of the free hormone out of the cell (Schell-Frederick and Dumont, 1970; Nadler, 1971). An elucidation of the effect of calcium on this somewhat unique secretory process could help to pinpoint its mode of action on the secretory mechanism.

At this point it is difficult to draw any definite conclusions concerning the role of calcium in thyroid function. Removal of calcium from the medium, or the addition of high concentrations of magnesium, only partially inhibits the TSH-induced release of thyroidal (^{131}I) iodine *in vitro* (Williams, 1972a), whereas the removal of sodium produces a more striking and rapid depression of TSH-stimulated ^{131}I release (Williams, 1972b). Such findings are in certain respects similar to those demonstrated in the salivary gland, where the effects of sodium deprivation rather than calcium lack are more readily demonstrable. But the observed effects of sodium deprivation on thyroid hormone secretion may only be a manifestation of changes in the calcium concentration of the follicular cell—a phenomenon already demonstrated in other tissues.

The action of calcium on the thyroid gland is made more complex by the fact that although calcium is not required for the TSH effect on colloid droplet formation, it appears to have actions on other aspects of thyroid cell function which can ultimately affect the amount of hormone released. Thus calcium is necessary for certain metabolic effects in the thyroid, most notably the increase in glucose oxidation attending TSH stimulation (Dekker and Field, 1970) and the increase in ^{32}P incorporation into phospholipids by TSH (Zor *et al.*, 1968). Moreover, calcium is needed for the TSH-stimulated transfer of ^{131}I from an intrathyroidal pool of iodine into thyroglobulin (Kondo and Ui, 1963). This latter effect of calcium—which is inhibited by magnesium—is not observed in a cell-free system, suggesting that the action of calcium is not due to a direct effect on the iodinating enzyme system but to an effect on the structure of the intact cell.

These studies certainly point to a general role for calcium in the secretory process of the follicular cell, and undoubtedly it is due, in part, to an action on general metabolic functions of the cell. However, an *in vitro* study by Williams suggests a possible dependence of thyroid secretory function on intracellular calcium (Williams, 1972a), which is analogous to that proposed for the action of ACTH on the adrenocortical cell (Jaanus and Rubin, 1971). The membrane events accompanying thyrotropin stimulation are also in harmony with such a conclusion. Thus, just as in the adrenal cortex, the trophic hormone—in this case TSH as well as excess potassium (Woodbury and Woodbury, 1963; Williams, 1966, 1970)—can induce changes in the membrane potential of the thyroid; but the depolarizing activity of potassium does not trigger thyroid hormone release, nor does it affect the releasing activity of TSH (Williams, 1972b). These data suggest either that a fall in membrane resistance is not the primary action of the pituitary trophic hormone or that if an increase in cell permeability is related to stimulatory activity then it is not the sole effect produced by stimulation. The dissociation between membrane events and the secretory response may be related to the fact that hormone stores are located extracellularly in the thyroid gland and are essentially lacking in the adrenal cortex. The absence of preformed intracellular hormone may require that the trophic hormone exert its effects through intracellular rather than extracellular calcium.

Of course up to now we have not as yet considered the role of cyclic AMP, and there is little doubt that in both the thyroid and adrenal cortex it plays some intermediary role in hormone action which culminates in the release response. The participation of cyclic AMP in the secretory mechanism will be considered in the final chapter, but it should be stated at this juncture that in the secretory systems where cyclic AMP appears to be an intermediate, calcium is also critically implicated. However, in these systems hormone stimulation does not appear to be associated with gross changes in cell membrane permeability, but with more specific and localized changes in calcium distribution. The thyroid follicular cell and adrenocortical cell are two prime examples of this situation. By contrast, in the adrenal chromaffin cell—where evidence for a role for cyclic AMP has yet to be established—membrane stimulation is associated with transmembrane ion fluxes. Thus at present it is not possible to explain the ubiquitous action of calcium in all secretory systems in terms of the Douglas concept of "stimulus–secretion coupling"; this concept may have to be modified in those systems where the role of cyclic AMP occurs in concert with that of calcium.

Furthermore, the question still remains unanswered as to whether the action of calcium on the secretory responses of the thyroid follicular cell and adrenocortical cell represents a direct effect on the secretory mechanism of these endocrine cells. This is a crucial problem to be solved, for if, indeed, future studies demonstrate that calcium also regulates the secretory processes in the thyroid and adrenal cortex, the ubiquity of the calcium effects will be extended to two systems which appear to have seemingly singular mechanisms for releasing their hormone, which do not involve exocytosis. Although the evidence so far suggests that stimulation of these two endocrine cells depends on a redistribution of cell calcium, we are still not able to answer the critical question whether the principal site of calcium action in secretory systems is solely confined to mechanisms involved with the discharge of the contents of the secretory granules of a cell or whether the action of calcium is much more basic and transcends the nature of the secretory process.

Pituitary Trophic Hormones

The anterior pituitary gland in some ways presents a similar picture to that painted for the adrenal medulla, although an elucidation of the sequence of events which occurs in this tissue is obscured by its functional and morphological heterogeneity. The anterior pituitary, a nonnervous tissue, contains at least six major hormones, each of which is sequestered within secretory organelles in a characteristic type of cell. Most, if not all, of the hormones of the anterior pituitary are activated by stimulating factors of hypothalamic origin (Schally *et al.*, 1973). However, despite the fact that stimuli for the release of anterior pituitary hormones *in vivo* are not neural and depolarization might not be a consequence of these stimuli, excess potassium is able to stimulate the release *in vitro* of growth hormone, luteinizing hormone, adrenocorticotropin, thyrotropin, and follicle-stimulating hormone (Geschwind, 1970). Only prolactin release is not readily augmented by high potassium (Parsons, 1970), which suggests that prolactin release is unaffected by the degree of polarization of the cell membrane. On the other hand, the inability of excess potassium to stimulate prolactin release *in vitro* may be due to the fact that prolactin release may already be near maximal levels due to the removal of a hypothalamic inhibitory factor. Although it would seem only logical to assume that potassium exerts its effects by depolarization, Milligan and Kraicer (1970) have demonstrated not just a depolarization but even a reversal of the transmembrane potential in anterior pituitary cells in the presence of 25 mM potassium.

Although such data provide us with some information as to the mechanism of action of a nonspecific depolarizing agent such as potassium, they do not enlighten us as to the mechanism of action of the hypothalamic stimulating principles, which are presumed to be the physiological stimuli. And indeed the effects of optimum concentrations of potassium and hypothalamic extract are, under certain conditions, additive (Samli and Geschwind, 1968), suggesting that both stimuli are promoting release by different mechanisms, although it may only indicate that hypothalamic releasing factors have functions in addition to effecting membrane depolarization. Yet the fact that both types of stimulation require the presence of calcium (Geschwind, 1969, 1970) and are inhibited by excess magnesium (Wakabayashi *et al.*, 1969; Parsons, 1970) might suggest that they both utilize the same final common pathway in the secretory process, although the triggering mechanisms may be different.

The mere demonstration of a reduction in hormone output when a tissue is incubated in a calcium-free solution does not allow one to conclude that calcium-free media inhibit secretion simply by preventing calcium influx into the cells. In fact, in some studies the very rigorous procedures used to rid the system of calcium, such as the use of chelating agents, may remove calcium not only from the extracellular milieu but also from intracellular sites. Experiments using radiocalcium may provide some information as to the locus of the critical calcium fraction; and indeed they have demonstrated an increase in the radiocalcium tissue space associated with growth hormone secretion induced by a purified growth hormone releasing factor, or by excess potassium (Milligan and Kraicer, 1970, 1972); but these experiments do not provide clear evidence as to whether this increased calcium space is due to an enhanced uptake of calcium from the extracellular fluid (increase in calcium influx) or a redistribution of cell calcium which causes a slowing of calcium efflux. Until the electrophysiological changes associated with stimulation by a purified hypothalamic releasing factor are known, it cannot be stated with any degree of certainty whether, under physiological conditions, influx of extracellular calcium or its cellular redistribution is the primary event in triggering the release response in the adenohypophysis.

Although the pivotal role of calcium in the secretory mechanism of preformed hormone from the anterior pituitary gland has been established, calcium may also be required for the synthesis of adenohypophyseal hormones. There is substantial evidence that an increase in adenohypophyseal hormone synthesis—as measured by an increase in total bioassayable hormone—occurs after administration of hypothalamic releasing factors *in vivo* or *in vitro* (Geschwind, 1969, 1970). The critical question in this regard, which cannot be answered at this time, is whether calcium involvement in the synthesis of follicle-stimulating hormone, for example, is a secondary phenomenon resulting from release or whether it is a process induced directly by the hypothalamic principle or excess potassium. Some insight into this aspect of calcium action may be obtained by noting that there is some evidence to suggest that calcium is involved in the biosynthesis of certain of the adenohypophyseal hormones (Jutisz and Paloma delaLlosa,

1970; MacLeod and Fontham, 1970) but not others (Samli and Geschwind, 1968).

However, whatever the specific locus of calcium action in the anterior pituitary gland, it is not at the general level of protein synthesis; for, unlike the adrenal cortex, inhibition of protein synthesis in the adenohypophysis on the whole does not interfere with hormone release, and amino acid incorporation into protein can proceed in a normal manner in the absence of calcium (Geschwind, 1969). In the adrenal cortex the protein synthesis required for ACTH-induced steroid synthesis and release appears to depend on the presence of calcium (Farese, 1971), which indicates that in this secretory organ one site of calcium action may be at the level of protein synthesis.

Geschwind (1970) has discussed some possibilities for the action of calcium on the energy-requiring secretory mechanism of the adenohypophysis. They include (1) to dissociate a hormone–carrier protein complex, (2) to produce a conformational change in the macromolecules of the granule and plasma membranes, (3) to activate a membrane phospholipase, (4) to promote adhesion of the secretory granule and the cell membrane, (5) to alter the colloidal state of the cytosol, (6) to release the inhibition of a myosin-like ATPase, and (6) to activate a protein kinase. But whatever the nature of calcium's role, the irregular effects produced by sodium and potassium deficiency (Wakabayashi *et al.*, 1969; MacLeod and Fontham, 1970; Parsons, 1970) and by ouabain (Geschwind, 1969) indicate that neither of these ions nor Na^+-K^+-activated ATPase is directly involved in regulating the release process of the adenohypophysis.

More careful consideration of these possibilities will be reserved for a subsequent chapter; however, it appears valid to conclude from the data so far accumulated from studies on the adenohypophysis, but even more strikingly on the thyroid and adrenal cortex, that stimulation of the target endocrine cell by its trophic hormone may not necessarily be associated with transmembrane ion fluxes resulting from nonspecific permeability changes. This is not to mitigate the importance of calcium in the mechanism of stimulus–secretion coupling but only to indicate that the locus of the calcium may emanate from a cellular site as well as from an extracellular site and that the action of the stimulating hormone may be to cause a specific cellular redistribution of this critical calcium fraction. We will have more to say to this point in the chapter on cyclic AMP.

Parathyroid Hormone and Calcitonin

Parathyroid hormone (PTH) and calcitonin—the latter secreted from the C cells of the thyroid gland—are two hormones which play a critical role in maintaining calcium homeostasis within the living organism. The significance of PTH in calcium homeostasis has long been recognized, since removal of parathyroid glands leads to a fall in calcium levels in plasma, tetany, and death (Copp, 1970). Although the administration of calcitonin lowers plasma calcium levels, the removal of the thyroid gland in mammals produces no changes in calcium levels, which suggests that this hormone exerts more of a modulating role in calcium metabolism. One site of action of these two hormones is bone, where PTH stimulates mobilization of calcium and calcitonin inhibits this process. PTH also affects calcium turnover at the level of the kidney, as evidenced by the finding that it stimulates calcium influx into the kidney cell in tissue culture (Borle, 1971).

Although PTH and calcitonin modulate calcium metabolism, their rate of release is in turn governed by the calcium concentration of the extracellular fluid which these hormones function to control. Patt and Luckhardt (1942) provided perhaps the first real demonstration that the concentration of ionized calcium in blood directly controls the rate of PTH secretion by perfusing calcium-depleted blood through an isolated dog thyroid–parathyroid gland. The injection of the perfusate into a second dog produced an increase in blood calcium which was similar to that obtained with parathyroid extract. Later, Sherwood et al., (1968), using more direct measurements of PTH by means of radioimmunoassay, confirmed that the rate of parathyroid secretion is rapidly responsive to changes in blood calcium. Perfusion of isolated parathyroid glands with calcium-deprived solution augments parathyroid hormone release, and the amount of hormone secreted bears a simple linear inverse relation to the plasma calcium concentration (Fig. 14).

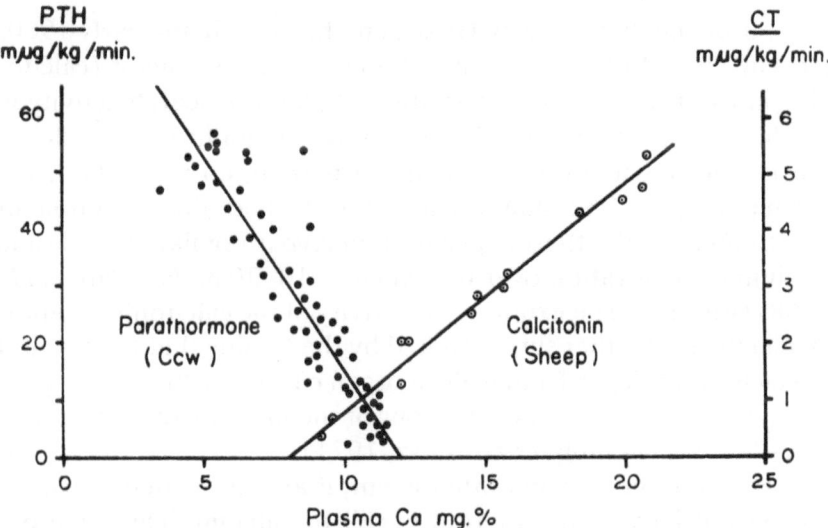

Fig. 14. Effect of the plasma calcium concentration on the secretory rate of parathormone in the cow and of calcitonin in an adult sheep (Copp, 1969).

In attempting to explain the anomalous effects of calcium in parathyroid secretion, one must seriously consider the possibility that biosynthesis of hormone may be the limiting factor in determining its rate of secretion, and calcium may exert its effect at this level. The evidence supporting this notion makes this possibility a very viable one (Sherwood *et al.*, 1968). Thus after an increase in the plasma calcium concentration, it may take 25 min for the concentration of circulating parathyroid hormone to decrease by 50%, which suggests that the calcium is not simply turning off a release mechanism. Conversely, after starting infusion of a calcium-chelating agent, such as EDTA, an increase in parathyroid hormone secretion occurs within 3–5 min, which is rather rapid; however, with a maintained EDTA infusion for 24 hr or more, there is a sustained high rate of secretion. This finding certainly indicates that to maintain the high rate of secretion the hormone supply has to be replenished by active hormone synthesis. Such studies *in vivo* are corroborated by studies *in vitro* showing that calcium can indeed regulate the rate of parathyroid hormone synthesis (Hamilton and Cohn, 1969).

After the discovery by Hirsch and Munson in the early 1960s (cf. Hirsch and Munson, 1969) of a hypocalcemic factor (calcitonin) in extracts of mammalian thyroid gland, research activity in this field has proliferated. The physiological significance of calcitonin is attested to by the fact that it is secreted throughout the normal range of plasma calcium levels, and the secretion of calcitonin from the thyroid perfused *in vivo* is regulated by plasma calcium concentration over the range of 10–20 mg% (Care *et al.*, 1968) (Fig. 14). The exquisite sensitivity of the calcitonin receptor mechanism is further substantiated by the finding that the amount of calcitonin release from cells in organ culture is directly proportional to the calcium concentrations of the medium over the range of 1–2.5 mM (Feinblatt and Raisz, 1971).

It is not known what other agent, if any, is needed to trigger the responsivity of the thyroid C cell to calcium. The secretory response induced by small changes in the calcium concentration apparently does not require intact innervation or the mediation of other glands. If indeed calcitonin release induced by calcium does not require any other stimulating agent, this would represent a rather unique system, since with other glands some prior stimulation is required to initiate the activity of calcium on the secretory process.

Stimulation may not be required for calcitonin release because either the calcium-active site is readily accessible from the extracellular fluid or calcium can readily penetrate into the cell without any additional permeability changes. The increase in calcitonin release in response to hypercalcemia is rapid but not immediate—occurring within 5 min. This may suggest that calcium manifests its stimulatory effects, at least in part, by enhancing hormone synthesis. The increased release of calcitonin observed with magnesium concentrations of 2–6 mM/liter may also be explained on the basis of an enhancement of hormone biosynthesis (Care *et al.*, 1971b). However, at higher magnesium concentrations, calcium-stimulated calcitonin secretion is profoundly inhibited. Thus the stimulatory effect of magnesium on the synthesis of calcitonin may be masked by its inhibitory effect on the release process.

CONCLUSIONS

This concludes the general survey of the various secretory systems where the role of calcium has been investigated. Because of the wide scope of the discussion, only what was deemed as the most salient information was included, but all of the evidence points to a key regulatory role for calcium in the events which lead to the extrusion of substances from cells. Calcium appears to act by transmitting the signal given by membrane recognition of the stimulus to some critical site within the cell. Many secretogogues—whether they be chemical or electrical—initiate the events in the secretory process by an action on the plasma membrane, which results in an increase in membrane permeability leading to an influx of extracellular calcium. Such a mechanism is likely to exist in electrically excitable tissue and the adrenal medulla.

However, evidence was also presented which supports the concept that a primary interaction of physiological and pharmacological stimulants with the receptors of certain target secretory cells somehow brings about the redistribution of cell calcium. The effect of secretogogues which act at some intracellular site would of course be mediated through the redistribution of cell calcium. However, it is too simplistic to generalize that the site of the critical calcium fraction is always extracellular when the action of the secretogogue is at the level of the cell membrane and intracellular when the secretogogue acts intracellularly, for ACTH and TSH—which are thought to act on the plasmalemma of their respective target cells—can also effect a translocation of cell calcium. Insulin release from the endocrine pancreas may also primarily involve the interaction of glucose with the β-cell membrane, but associated with a shift in calcium from some cellular pool.

Thus at present it is not possible to provide a clear explanation of the events involved in the "stimulus" aspect of "stimulus–secretion coupling" in all systems; however, whatever the locus of the critical calcium fraction, a comparison of data from a variety of organs shows that the translocation of calcium produced by chemical or electrical stimulation is responsible for activating the release mechanisms of a wide variety of secretory systems which extrude a large number of diverse substances. A discussion of the nature of the molecular events by which the redistribution of calcium through the various extra- and intracellular compartments culminates in the extrusion of secretory product will be reserved for the next chapter.

CHAPTER 3

The Nature of the Role of Calcium in Secretion

MECHANISM OF SECRETION

In considering the nature of calcium's action in the secretory process, one must first ascertain how the secretory product is transferred from the site of storage to the extracellular fluid. Since endocrine tissues are much easier to study by biochemical methods than nervous tissue, it has been possible to define the nature of the secretory process in certain endocrine organs with the aid of advanced biochemical and morphological techniques. Studies employing such techniques have established that hormones in most glands are stored in membrane-bound granules, so it seems reasonable to consider that the secretory granules are not just inert stores of hormone but play an active role in secreting the hormones from the cell.

The particulate fraction harboring the stored hormone has been isolated from a number of endocrine tissues by differential centrifugation and its properties studied *in vitro*. The catecholamine-containing granule fraction of the adrenal medulla has perhaps undergone the most extensive investigation. The chromaffin granules are characterized by a remarkably high content of catecholamine (20% of dry weight), adenine nucleotide—mainly ATP—(15% of dry weight), and protein (35% of dry weight) (Hillarp, 1959). The protein has some enzymatic activities, which include ATPase, dopamine β-hydroxylase, and cytochrome $b559$, although there is also a high concentration of nonenzymatic water-soluble protein (Winkler, 1971). Sulfated mucopolysaccharides can also be identified (Fillion et al., 1971; Margolis and Margolis, 1973), and they may aid in the binding and storage of the amine. The calcium content of the chromaffin granules is very high for a soft-tissue fraction, having six times as much calcium per gram protein as do rat liver mitochondria (Borowitz et al., 1965). Although catecholamine and ATP present in the chromaffin granules are probably bound to macromolecular components and are metabolically and osmotically inactive, calcium appears to be turning over, as indicated by the finding that after infusion of radiocalcium into the isolated perfused adrenal gland the isotope can be found concentrated in the chromaffin granules as well as in the mitochondria (Borowitz, 1970; Winkler et al., 1972). This mechanism for sequestering calcium may provide the means whereby the physiological activity of calcium is terminated in many secretory cells.

Although most of the medullary catecholamine is found in the particulate fraction after tissue homogenization and differential centrifugation, approximately 20% is usually present in the supernatant. Whether this represents an extragranular store of amine reflecting the presence of a small pool of newly synthesized catecholamine in the cytosol or is artifactual as a consequence of the isolation procedures has not been definitely determined (Smith and Winkler, 1972). However, whether or not an extragranular store actually exists, it does not directly participate in the release process, for by studying the release of other components of the granule it has been possible to identify the mechanism by which catecholamine leaves the cell as exocytosis, that is, fusion of the granule membrane with the plasma membrane.

The elucidation of the nature of secretory mechanisms began with the elegant work of the late Nils-Äke Hillarp and his associates, in Sweden. They found that when adrenals were stimulated in vivo with insulin or morphine, there was a parallel fall in the concentration of catecholamine and nucleotide, such that the molar ratio of amines to nucleotides was not markedly changed (Carlsson *et al.*, 1957). However, when a search was made for nucleotides or their breakdown products in the gland there were none to be found (Hillarp, 1960). This might suggest that other granule constituents, in addition to the hormone, are extruded after stimulation. A few years later, Douglas and his associates demonstrated that not only was adenine nucleotide released into the cat adrenal perfusate after medullary stimulation by a variety of agents (Douglas, 1968) but also the molar ratio of catecholamine to ATP and its catabolites in the perfusate was 4.2, which is very close to the value of the molar ratio in the cat adrenal (3.7) (Hillarp and Thieme, 1959). This study established that the chromaffin granule was the immediate source of the catecholamine secreted from the gland.

About the same time, Banks and Helle (1965) reported that the perfused bovine adrenal also secretes protein following stimulation. The protein, which is only one of eight soluble proteins, was purified and given the name "chromogranin" by Blaschko *et al.* (1967). It gave a precipitate with an antiserum prepared against protein purified from bovine chromaffin granules. Kirshner and his associates confirmed the identification and characterization of chromogranin by complement-fixation techniques and showed that the catecholamines and chromogranins were released from the isolated adrenal in the same relative amounts as those found in the intact chromaffin granule (Kirshner *et al.*, 1967; see also Kirshner and Kirshner, 1971) (Fig. 15). The physiological significance of these results was strengthened by the finding of Blaschko *et al.* (1967) that the ratio of catecholamine to chromogranin in the calf adrenal venous blood after splanchnic stimulation *in vivo* was similar to that of the soluble lysate of chromaffin granules. Other constituents of the chromaffin granules, including soluble dopamine β-hydroxylase (Kirshner and Viveros, 1970), sulfated mucopolysaccharides (Margolis *et al.*, 1973), and calcium (Rubin *et al.*, 1967), are also released *pari passu* with medullary catecholamine. On the other hand, adrenal stimulation is not associated with a release of extragranular protein. Soluble enzymes, such as tyrosine hydroxylase and lactic dehydrogenase,

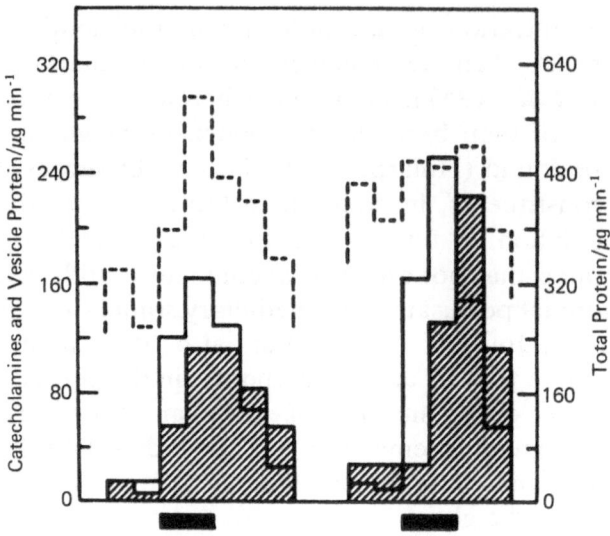

Fig. 15. Concomitant secretion of catecholamines and chromogranin A from perfused bovine adrenal glands. Catecholamines, open bars; total protein, broken line; chromogranin A, shaded bars (Kirshner *et al.*, 1967).

have a much smaller molecular diameter than chromogranin, so if release occurs by diffusion of the granular components through the cytoplasm, then one might expect cytoplasmic substances to also be released; but they are not (Smith and Winkler, 1972).

The concept that release occurs by extrusion of the whole granule was proposed long ago by Cramer (1928) as a likely mechanism of secretion. But the advancement of present-day biochemical techniques enables one to rule out such a possibility, for whereas the soluble components of the granule are recovered in the perfusate the insoluble products are retained in the gland (Smith and Winkler, 1972). Thus the chromaffin granule also contains phospholipids and cholesterol, and these lipids are presumed to be present in the plasma membrane. After stimulation of the gland, only very small increases in the amounts of phospholipids and cholesterol are found in the perfusate. In the rabbit 50% of the dopamine hydroxylase activity is also in the insoluble residue, and there is no change in enzyme content associated with the particulate fraction of the cell homogenates after insulin stimulation, although there is a decrease in the soluble dopamine hydroxylase content of the gland (Kirshner and Viveros, 1970).

All of the biochemical evidence accumulated from the comprehensive studies—all too briefly described—indicates that medullary catecholamine release occurs by the process of exocytosis. Actually, DeRobertis and Vaz Ferreira (1957) first proposed exocytosis as a mechanism for catecholamine release on the basis of electron microscopic studies, but it was Coupland (1965) who first obtained clear pictures showing continuity of two interacting membranes. Diner (see Grynszpan-Winograd, 1971), by careful analysis of many sections, provided more unequivocal evidence of granules adhering to, or fusing with, plasma membranes from hamster glands (Fig. 16). However, similar analysis of adrenal sections from other animals by the same investigator failed to support her findings in the hamster.

Even if one is willing to focus only on the positive findings of Diner, one must question whether the micrographs depicting the interaction of the secretory granule and cell membrane are related to the process of secretion or whether they are merely random events. But the use of the freeze-etching technique, which allows for a better visualization of the cell surface, has also provided morphological evidence in support of medullary secretion by exocytosis (Smith et al., 1973). Although even the most avid electron microscopist would agree that purely morphological observations do not allow an elucidation of the secretory process, such findings do provide circumstantial evidence in support of the more conclusive biochemical data favoring exocytosis as the mechanism of medullary secretion.

The similarity between the factors governing release of catecholamine from adrenal chromaffin cells and neurohumors from peripheral nerves was clearly demonstrated by the studies enumerated in the previous chapter. This might lead one to consider whether neurotransmitter release also occurs by exocytosis. Norepinephrine, as well as acetylcholine, is contained in membrane-limited structures known as synaptic vesicles. These vesicles are much smaller than secretory granules found in the adrenal medulla or in other endocrine organs, and electron microscopic evidence in support of the idea of secretion by

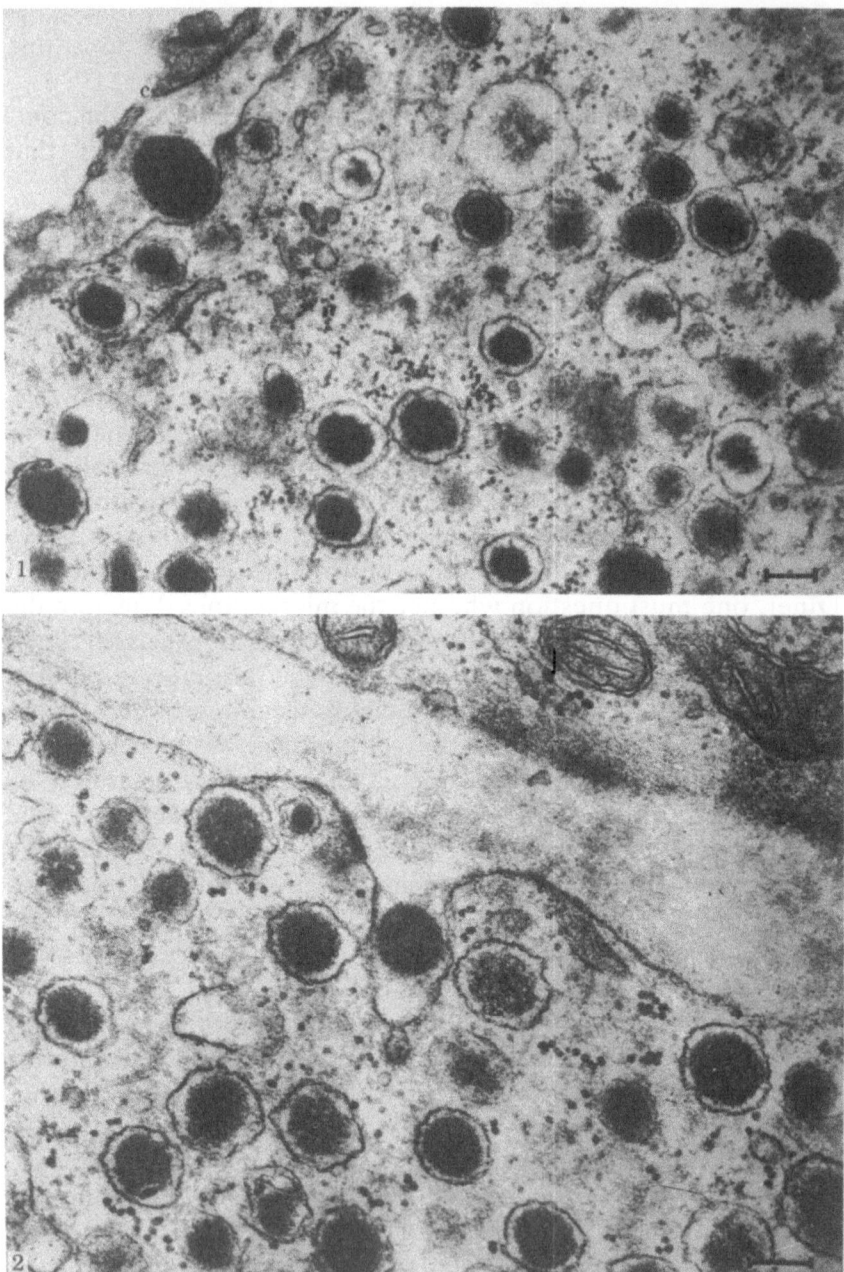

Fig. 16. Exocytosis in the adrenal medulla of the hamster
(Grynszpan-Winograd, 1971).

exocytosis is difficult to obtain in these neuronal tissues (Fillenz, 1971). However, indirect evidence supports this concept. Thus neurophysiological studies seem to indicate that neuronal norepinephrine is released in discrete multimolecular packets by a process which requires calcium (Smith and Winkler, 1972). Moreover, pharmacological studies which utilize the action of reserpine in preventing the uptake of catecholamines from the cytosol into the granule have shown that the norepinephrine diverted from its granule store to the cytoplasm by the effects of reserpine cannot be released by nerve stimulation. On the other hand, tyramine, whose amine-releasing activity from the adrenergic neuron does not appear to require the presence of calcium, can release cytoplasmic norepinephrine (Chubb *et al.*, 1972). Such evidence points to the fact that the fundamental action of calcium is intimately involved with the process of exocytosis (Smith and Winkler, 1972).

Biochemical studies also support this concept. ATP release from adrenergic nerves cannot be studied, since, unlike chromaffin tissue, its presence in the catecholamine-containing vesicles isolated from neurons represents only a very small fraction of the total amount in tissue; however, protein release from peripheral adrenergic organs has been demonstrated after nerve stimulation. Moreover, the protein released has been identified by immunodiffusion techniques and complement fixation as chromogranin (Geffen *et al.*, 1970; Smith, 1971). Nerve stimulation also leads to enhanced release of dopamine hydroxylase, as long as calcium is present, but soluble enzymes such as tyrosine hydroxylase and dopa decarboxylase are not released (cf. Smith, 1971; Johnson *et al.*, 1971).

Thus although certain differences between the splenic nerve granule fraction and the chromaffin granule fraction have been uncovered, such as the fact that ATP concentrations are much lower in the nerve granule fraction whereas the dopamine hydroxylase content is relatively much higher, the data obtained from cation studies and biochemical analyses of tissue effluent indicate that they are probably only quantitative differences and are not a manifestation of a qualitatively different process (Lagercrantz, 1971). It is probable that catecholamine release both from adrenal chromaffin cells and from sympathetic nerves occurs through a process of exocytosis in which calcium plays a crucial role.

In order to ascertain whether exocytosis might be common to the release of other neurotransmitters, we next explore what evidence exists in its favor regarding acetylcholine release. It was established from studies in cholinergic nerves by Katz and his associates that when the calcium concentration is low enough, or the magnesium concentration high, the end-plate potential is reduced to a minimal amplitude and becomes identical in size and shape to the spontaneously occurring miniature end-plate potentials (Katz, 1958). It was proposed that the miniature end-plate potential represents the release of acetylcholine in discrete molecular packets or quanta and that the end-plate potential consists of a summation of such quanta. At about the same time, electron microscopic studies established that large numbers of small membrane-limited vesicles were concentrated in the nerve ending (DeRobertis and Bennett, 1955). They were believed to be the storage particles for acetylcholine and therefore to represent morphological quantal units. Although there is as yet no irrefutable biochemical or morphological evidence which unequivocally demonstrates that the vesicle represents the locus of acetylcholine storage, most experts in this field feel that this is most certainly the case. For example, Katz (1971) states that "The fact that experimental alterations of the surface membrane induce very large changes in the frequency of discharge, but not in the size of the quantal packet, favors the concept of intracellular prepackaging, which indicates transmitter is parceled in synaptic vesicles."

If the vesicles represent the site of storage for acetylcholine, and quantal release is related to the presence of neurotransmitter in these vesicles, then one might expect that stimulation and release of acetylcholine would be associated with alterations in the number of synaptic vesicles; and indeed there have been reports of a fall in the number of vesicles after nerve stimulation (Jones and Kwanbunbumpen, 1970), or in the presence of excess potassium (Hubbard and Kwanbunbumpen, 1968) or black widow spider venom (Longenecker et al., 1970). In addition, procedures that accelerate or depress the synthesis or release of acetylcholine by rat diaphragm seem to cause noticeable changes in the vesicles situated close to the synaptic membrane (Jones and Kwanbun-bumpen, 1970). On the other hand, an increase in the number of cholinergic vesicles present has been reported to occur after splanchnic nerve stimulation (DeRobertis, 1959). The apparent problems associated with correlating vesicle and neuronal activity may be related to the fact that only a small fraction (circa 20%) of the total acetylcholine store is available for release, so that any change in granule vesicle population may be localized rather than diffuse. Furthermore, newly synthesized acetylcholine is released before it equilibrates with preformed stores, so that releasable transmitter is replaced partly by synthesis as well as by mobilization of the preformed acetylcholine store (Collier, 1969). The replenishment of acetylcholine stores by synthesis would of course curtail the decrease in the tissue acetylcholine content, and possibly in the number of vesicles.

Despite the absence of really definitive evidence to support the concept that acetylcholine is released from vesicles by exocytosis, the quantal hypothesis as originally proposed by Katz and his associates has gained general acceptance. This concept has achieved favor because not only have miniature end-plate potentials been observed at the neuromuscular junction but miniature postsynaptic potentials are also demonstrable in certain sympathetically innervated smooth muscle preparations (Kuriyama, 1964) and at central synapses (cf. Colomo and Erulkar, 1968), all of which support the idea that the synaptic vesicles represent the quantum subcellular unit of neurotransmitter.

If one accepts the concept that the readily releasable store of acetylcholine is the synaptic vesicle, then one can make a legitimate case for the idea that release does occur by exocytosis on the basis of some morphological and biochemical evidence which, though not nearly as conclusive as that obtained on the sympathetic system, does tend to support this idea. Thus exocytosis appears to have been demonstrated by Nickel and Potter (1971) by the freeze-etching technique in the electric tissue of *Torpedo*, while in the rat nerve–muscle preparation Musick and Hubbard (1972) observed a concomitant release of protein along with acetylcholine after nerve stimulation. This finding suggests that the release of this neurotransmitter does not occur by simple diffusion, but supports the idea that acetylcholine release is accompanied by the release of other vesicular constituents and represents a similar phenomenon to that occurring in the adrenal medulla and sympathetic neuron. However, much more evidence is still needed to substantiate the tentative hypothesis that acetylcholine release occurs by exocytosis.

Although most morphologists would agree that it is quite difficult to demonstrate exocytosis by conventional electron microscopic techniques, there have been isolated reports of such evidence from a number of endocrine organs, such as the pancreas, adenohypophysis, and neurohypophysis, as well as the adrenal medulla (cf. Smith, 1972). The excellent morphological evidence for exocytosis obtained by Douglas and his associates (Douglas *et al.*, 1970) in the neurohypophysis is supported by biochemical evidence. The neural lobe of the mammalian pituitary gland is the site of storage and release of vasopressin and oxytocin, and 50–80% of these hormones are found within the so-called granular fraction closely associated with the binding protein, neurophysin (Dean and Hope, 1968). Evidence supporting exocytosis as the mechanism of secretion should show that the release of pituitary hormone is accompanied by the release of neurophysin, and indeed Fawcett *et al.* (1968) demonstrated in the intact dog that both vasopressin and neurophysin were secreted into the circulation in response to hemorrhage. Moreover, these same investigators found that after labeling of protein (both hormone and neurophysin) *in vivo*, glands subsequently incubated *in vitro* and challenged with excess potassium simultaneously released both vasopressin and neurophysin. This important finding has been corroborated by Uttenthal *et al.* (1971) and by Friesen and coworkers (Cheng *et al.*, 1972) and has been elaborated to show that changes in the ionic millieu which alter the hormonal response to excess potassium will produce the same effects on the release of neurophysin. Thus the presence of calcium in the medium is critical for the release of neurophysin (Fig. 17), whereas in the absence of sodium the release of binding protein is not depressed, but may even be enhanced. Magnesium, which depresses the release of vasopressin induced by high potassium, also blocks the release of neurophysin. These findings, which demonstrate that factors which

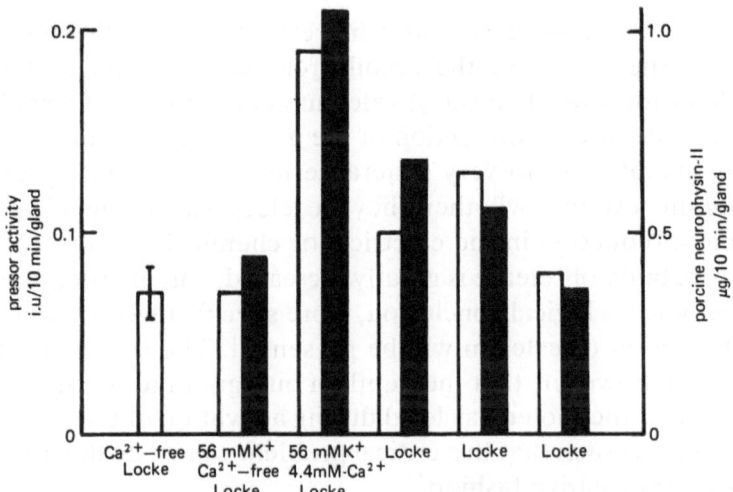

Fig. 17. Release of vasopressin and neurophysin II from isolated porcine neurohypophyses in response to excess potassium. Open bars show pressor activity, blocked bars the amount of neurophysin in samples of the incubation medium containing various calcium concentrations (Uttenthal *et al.*, 1971).

stimulate or inhibit the release of vasopressin have the same effect on the release of neurophysin, add strong support for the idea of secretion by exocytosis. Such evidence minimizes the possibility—which has been given some consideration—that calcium entering the nerve ending following depolarization frees *extragranular* hormone from its binding with neurophysin, and the free hormone diffuses out of the cell (Ginsburg, 1968). The finding that there is a greater release of hormone than of neurophysin after stimulation could be explained on the basis of some release occurring through a process not involving exocytosis; another possible explanation for this disparity is that secretion may occur by exocytosis from a specific population of granules having a high hormone/neurophysin ratio (Pickup *et al.*, 1973).

MODE OF CALCIUM ACTION

While the dependence of neurotransmitter or hormone release on storage of preformed material is by no means proven, the conclusion which emerges from the evidence adduced so far is that the secretory product is stored in vesicles or granules and this provides the source of the readily releasable product. Thus in searching for a mechanism of calcium action one must somehow implicate it with an interaction of the granule membrane and the plasma membrane. In very general terms, one may interpret the membrane events—whether they be electrical or chemical—as causing a reduction in the electrical or chemical barriers, so that the probability of release is greatly increased. But in order to carry this story to its logical conclusion, more specific theories concerning the action of calcium will be presented. The reader must be cautioned, however, that the depth of our ignorance of the events occurring at the molecular level during activation of the secretory mechanism is such that this critical problem can be dealt with only in a very speculative fashion.

Physical Theories

In viewing the secretory process as electrical events, it has been suggested that vesicles or granules, like the cell membrane, are charged and are either attracted to or repelled by electrostatic forces. The medullary chromaffin granules (Matthews *et al.*, 1972) and polypeptide-containing granules from the neurohypophysis (Poisner and Douglas, 1968) appear to bear a net negative charge (as determined by electrophoretic mobility) and would in the resting state be repelled by the fixed negative charges on the cell membrane. Calcium entry could augment release by neutralizing the negative charges of the chromaffin granule and thereby expedite the interaction of the granule membrane and plasmalemma (Blioch *et al.*, 1968; Hubbard, 1970). The hypothesis that charge neutralization plays a role in hormone release, and that the ability of other ions to replace calcium in the release process simply depends on the valence of a given ion, does not hold up under careful scrutiny, for magnesium (which is an inhibitor of the release process), like calcium, causes a neutralization of the negative charges of the granules *in vitro* (Banks, 1966). The acetylcholine-containing vesicles—like the chromaffin granules—also appear to be charged, although the sign of the charge is a matter of dispute. In fact, there is some evidence to indicate that the acetylcholine-containing vesicles bear a net positive charge (Bass and Moore, 1966; Hubbard, 1970). But how the dispersal of the positive charges of the vesicle leads to an enhanced interaction with the axonal membrane has not been adequately explained, even in a most speculative fashion. Thus the charge neutralization theory has few experimental data to support its continued consideration.

Katz and his associates (Del Castillo and Katz, 1956) provided another way of envisaging the nature of the events in the release mechanism when they elaborated the quantal theory of acetylcholine release. They proposed that the synaptic vesicles are in constant random motion—perhaps due to thermal agitation—and bombard the terminal axonal membrane. Although the rate of collision between vesicles and plasma membrane is very high at all times, release occurs only in the improbable event of the interaction of the synaptic vesicle with the neuronal membrane. This event results in the opening of the vesicle to the extracellular fluid or synaptic space and leads to the release of transmitter. According to this model, the entry of calcium which occurs during membrane depolarization would increase the chance of vesicles interacting with the plasma membrane by increasing the number of sites where the vesicles can react with the membrane and thereby increase the amount of transmitter released. Under such circumstances, calcium may enhance release by decreasing the cytoplasmic viscosity of the cell. And indeed calcium and the other alkaline earths have rather similar effects on certain physicochemical properties of cell sap and will cause a decrease in cytoplasmic viscosity (Hodgkin and Katz, 1949b), induce gel formation (Heilbrunn, 1956), and even have the capacity to disrupt cytoplasmic granules (Gross, 1954). However, this appealing possibility is not supported by the morphological findings of Woodin *et al.* (1963), who observed that the effects of calcium on leucocidin-treated leukocytes were not related to any action on the cytoplasmic movements of the secretory granules, but to the subsequent stage of adherence of the granule to the cell membrane, which culminates in degranulation. This finding may represent a potentially very critical clue to as the nature of calcium's action, in light of the ability of calcium to promote membrane fusion reactions in a number of biological systems (see Poste and Allison, 1971). An enhancement of membrane fusion would also imply that calcium which enters the cell need not penetrate any further than the inner side of the cell membrane to exert its effect.

Chemical Theories

Although calcium can cause a rapid and explosive secretory response in such tissues as the adrenal medulla and endocrine pancreas, a delay (in milliseconds) has been noted between the onset of presynaptic depolarization and the arrival of acetylcholine at the frog postsynaptic membrane (Hubbard, 1970). This delay is almost all of presynaptic origin and may be accounted for by the increase in calcium entry and/or the changes induced by the entry of calcium. This may imply that calcium entry triggers a chemical reaction. The temperature dependence of the release process, which has been observed at cholinergic junctions (Hubbard, 1970) and with catecholamine release induced by cholinergic agents and high potassium in the perfused adrenal gland (Douglas and Rubin, unpublished observations), supports this assumption. Moreover, in all of the calcium-dependent secretory systems in which an energy requirement for secretion has been studied by the use of metabolic inhibitors, it appears as if energy is indeed required for maintaining secretion (Rubin, 1970; Geschwind, 1969, 1970). Furthermore, the activity of calcium as a secretogogue has been closely correlated with the ability of the tissue to produce metabolic energy, and a stoichiometric relation between the calcium and ATP concentration appears critical for monitoring the amount of hormone release (Rubin, 1970).

An energy-requiring chemical reaction would necessitate the splitting of ATP, and ATPase has been found in the membrane of secretory granules from a wide variety of cells (Douglas, 1968; Rubin, 1970). Moreover, ATP stimulates the release of hormone from isolated granule preparations suspended in media rich in sodium or potassium, and this releasing activity is inhibited by substances blocking the ATPase activity of the granules (Poisner, 1973).

Although ATP and ATPase can modulate the release of catecholamine and vasopressin from isolated granule preparations *in vitro*, calcium does not enhance significantly the release of secretory product from various isolated granule preparations (cf. Rubin, 1970). These findings suggest that if calcium and ATP interact to trigger secretion, a third factor, not present in isolated granule preparations, must be present in the intact gland; and it has been postulated that the activation of an extragranular ATPase may be instrumental in causing the granule to attach to the surface membrane (Douglas, 1968). Attaining an answer to this question is complicated by the fact that a number of different ATPases exist in secretory tissues. For example, chromaffin granules as well as mitochondrial and microsomal fractions of bovine adrenal medulla manifest ATPase activity, and the ATPase of each fraction is stimulated by calcium to a different degree (Banks, 1965). But despite the lack of direct evidence for its support, it appears worthwhile to present a model developed by Poisner and Trifaro (1967) (see also Poisner, 1970) which advances the concept that the interaction between ATP and ATPase, promoted *in situ* by calcium, brings about the attachment of the granule membrane to the plasmalemma. This leads to membrane fusion, *a resulting conformational change in the granule membrane,* and the release of the granule contents (Fig. 18). Although the model proposed by Poisner and Trifaro appears consistent with much of the existing evidence, caution must be employed in drawing conclusions from *in vitro* studies. The inability of calcium to augment hormone release from isolated granule preparations tells us that the effect of calcium in activating the release mechanism is not the result of a direct action on the secretory granule. On the other hand, the ability of ATP to enhance hormone release from isolated granules may be viewed in terms of a nonphysiological phenomenon if one favors the now well-accepted concept that the release response *in situ* involves not one, but two, membrane components—the granule membrane and the plasmalemma.

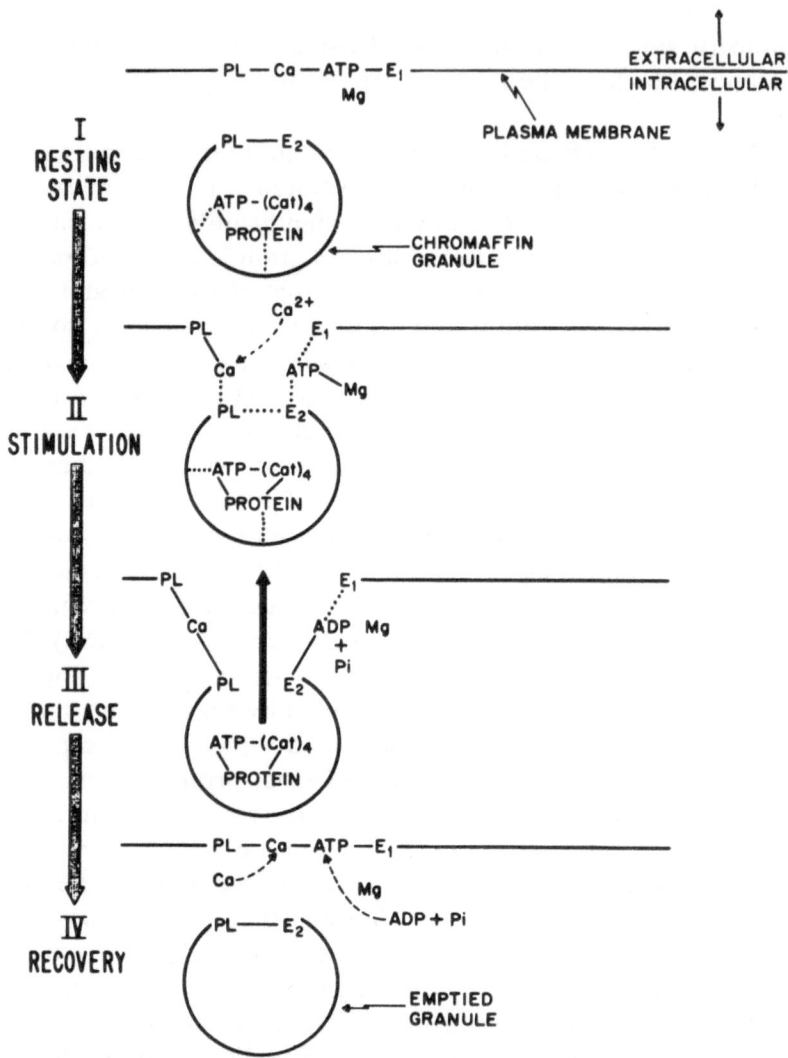

Fig. 18. A proposed model for catecholamine release from the adrenal medulla. On stimulation, calcium and ATP are freed from all membrane, permitting hydrolysis of ATP and influx of ions. Calcium forms a link between anionic groups in plasma membrane and membranes of chromaffin granules. The interaction between ATP and a site on the chromaffin granule membrane, which results in hydrolysis of ATP, produces some conformational change in the granule membrane, permitting the release of granule contents. Hydrolysis of ATP can occur by plasma membrane ATPase (E_1) or granule membrane ATPase (E_2). Restoration of initial condition involves resynthesis of ATP, rebinding of calcium by the plasma membrane, and return of granular membrane to its original state (Poisner and Trifaro, 1967).

MICROTUBULAR–MICROFILAMENTOUS SYSTEM

There is little doubt that clearer insight into the mechanism of calcium action would be afforded by a better understanding of the means by which the secretory granule reaches the cell membrane. One possible means would be a system of intercommunicating channels or tubules which would provide the pathway to the cell surface. Such a potential system was discovered at the turn of the century when the light microscope revealed, in silver-stained preparations of many kinds of nerve cells, thin fibrous structures which were called neurofibrils (cf. Wuerker and Kirkpatrick, 1972). The electron microscopist has further characterized these structures into microtubules and microfilaments. Microtubules appear to provide a structural framework to support cytoplasmic structures, and they are also a prime component of mitotic spindles, flagella, and cilia, which are all associated with kinesis. Microfilaments are thought to be composed of actin-like proteins, so that they may also serve to modulate cellular motility. The involvement of microtubular and microfilamentous systems in the nonrandom movement of substances within the cytoplasm may also include the migration of secretory granules. Calcium might act to facilitate granule transport, for example, by causing contraction of microtubules (Schmitt, 1968; Malaisse et al., 1971b). On the other hand, the microtubules may not manifest contractile properties but may merely provide a template for microfilament contraction which would elicit movement.

The original postulate proposed by Schmitt in 1968 of direct contact between cytoplasmic particles and microtubules provides an attractive explanation for the mechanism of secretory granule transport. Although the existence of microtubules in a wide variety of cells seems beyond dispute, the morphological evidence that this system represents a highly organized cytoskeleton which might be responsible for the migration of the secretory granules to the cell membrane is not at all convincing. Morphological studies reveal few, if any, microtubules at nerve endings where neurotransmitter release appears to occur, and only small numbers of microtubules have been observed in other secretory tissues; even when present, they may have no special orientation.

The involvement of the microtubular–microfilament system in the intracellular transport of secretory granules is based not only on its morphological demonstration but also on pharmacological studies which appear to indicate that agents that may have more or less specific effects on the microtubular–microfilamentous system of secretory cells will interfere with the release of many hormones. These agents include the alkaloids, colchicine and vinblastine, which bind to and disintegrate microtubules; heavy water (deuterium oxide), which inhibits microtubule function not by disrupting them but by hyperstabilizing them in a reversible manner; and cytochalasin B, a fungal metabolite which does not seem to affect the structure or function of microtubules but disrupts and even causes the disappearance of microfilaments.

The effects of these agents on the microtubules and microfilaments do not limit their actions to the secretory process. Thus the mitotic spindle which controls the migration of chromosomes during mitosis is composed of microtubules. Colchicine and vinblastine produce a decrease in the number and length of microtubules in the mitotic spindle and the eventual complete dissolution of these organelles, leading to an arrest of mitosis (Malawista, 1971). It has also been suggested that fast proximodistal axoplasmic transport of substances occurs through a mechanism related to microtubules, and in accord with this hypothesis local application of colchicine to an adrenergic nerve causes an accumulation of neurotransmitter and cell organelles proximal to the site of application (Dählstrom, 1970; Banks *et al.*, 1971).

Lacy *et al.* (1968) were the first to suggest that the microtubular–microfilamentous system might be involved in the mechanism of insulin release. They presented morphological evidence for the existence of the cell organelles in pancreatic islet cells and found that colchicine inhibits the secretion of insulin induced by glucose. Malaisse and his associates (Malaisse *et al.*, 1971b; Malaisse, 1972) corroborated and extended these findings to include other agents. However, certain discrepancies were observed (see Allison, 1973). Thus whereas vinblastine and deuterium oxide inhibited both the first and second phases of glucose-induced insulin secretion, colchicine inhibited only the second phase (Lacy *et al.*, 1972). Moreover, cytochalasin B, which disrupts microfilaments, does not inhibit but in fact enhances insulin release induced by glucose (Orci *et al.*, 1971). These data indicate that the effects of these agents vary within a given organ. And indeed this fact is supported by data obtained from other secretory systems. For example, although colchicine inhibits acetylcholine release from the frog neuromuscular junction (Hofmann *et al.*, 1973), cytochalasin and vinblastine have no discernible effect on this system (Katz, 1972). Moreover, deuterium oxide does not inhibit evoked catecholamine release from the perfused adrenal gland, but in fact enhances release (Poisner and Bernstein, 1971). In comparing the effects of these agents on various tissues, other discrepancies become manifest; although colchicine inhibits thyroid ^{131}I release (Temple *et al.*, 1972), it does not inhibit the release of pituitary thyrotropin or protein from the salivary gland and exocrine pancreas, and even stimulates the release of rat anterior pituitary hormones *in vitro* (Sundberg *et al.*, 1973). Deuterium oxide, while enhancing evoked medullary catecholamine secretion, inhibits insulin (Lacy *et al.*, 1972) and thyroid hormone secretion (Williams and Wolff, 1972). Do such data suggest that the contribution of microtubules to the secretory process differs from tissue to tissue, or do they imply that the primary action of colchicine and other so-called inhibitors of microtubules is not on microtubules at all?

The lack of effect of cytochalasin on insulin and acetylcholine release might indicate that the microfilaments play no direct role in the secretory mechanism, but this agent does inhibit the release of amylase from the rat parotid gland (Butcher and Goldman, 1972), histamine from mast cells (Gillespie *et al.*, 1968; Orr *et al.*, 1972), growth hormone and ACTH from the adenohypophysis (Kraicer and Milligan, 1971), and vasopressin from the neurohypophysis (Douglas and Sorimachi, 1972a). Thus if one accepts the very tenuous concept that all of these agents produce their principal effects by acting on the microtubules or microfilaments, it would be necessary to take into account the fact that the secretory processes in various tissues exhibit different responses to the agents which are presumed to interact with the microtubules or microfilaments, and these effects must be defined for each tissue. A further

possible—but rather implausible—explanation for these somewhat confusing findings is that the secretory processes may vary
from tissue to tissue. In any event, convincing evidence for a causal
relationship between the pharmacological effects on microtubules
and microfilaments and the impairment of exocytosis is still
lacking.

It is well known to the pharmacologist that chemical agents
are notorious for their nonspecificity of action, and it is apparent
that the actions of these inhibitors, especially in the high concentrations required in some systems to demonstrate effects, are not
confined to the microtubules or microfilaments but have other
demonstrable effects which could readily account for their actions
on secretion. Thus, in nerve, the concentration of colchicine
required to block the liberation of norepinephrine from adrenergic
nerve terminals by nicotine or high potassium is at least one
order of magnitude higher than that required to block axoplasmic transport (Sorimachi *et al.*, 1973). This makes it unlikely
that the inhibition of norepinephrine release by colchicine is a consequence of its interference with the structure and
function of microtubules. Interference of colchicine with
stimulus–secretion coupling could be explained by its interaction with the cell membrane. And indeed in perfused adrenal
glands colchicine and vinblastine block acetylcholine-
evoked catecholamine release without affecting—even enhancing—release evoked by excess potassium (Trifaro *et al.*,
1972). Similarly, cytochalasin B action may also be at the level of
the cholinergic receptor, since in perfused rabbit adrenal glands it
inhibits secretory responses to acetylcholine much more profoundly than responses to excess potassium (Douglas and Sorimachi,
1972b). The anticholinergic effects of colchicine have also been
demonstrated with glycoprotein secretion from the submaxillary
gland (Rossignol *et al.*, 1972). However, the idea that these agents
act as simple cholinergic antagonists in rat salivary glands is
mitigated by the recent findings that, in contrast to the receptor
antagonist, atropine, colchicine does not inhibit glycogen depletion, and vinblastine has no effect on increased calcium flux
induced by cholinergic stimulation (B. Rossignol, personal communication). These data suggest an intracellular site rather than
interaction at the receptor level, but whether these inhibitory

actions are related to effects on the microtubular system is still an unanswered question.

The diverse effects of an agent such as cytochalasin B would also indicate that caution must be employed in interpreting the results drawn from experiments employing these agents (Burnside and Manacek, 1972). Cytochalasin B exerts inhibitory effects on such varied cell functions as morphogenesis, cytokinesis, and phagocytosis (cf. Zigmond and Hirsch, 1972). Such widespread effects may be indicative of a more general depressant action, such as that observed with metabolic inhibitors. The relatively long latency of action of these agents (greater than 1 hr) would support such an assumption. Although biochemical studies indicate that cytochalasin B has no significant inhibitory action on certain cell metabolic activities, such as respiration or protein turnover, it does inhibit glucose transport and glycolysis in leukocytes and hepatoma cells (Zigmond and Hirsch, 1972; Estensen and Plagemann, 1972). So, while one would not infer that the principal effect of all of these agents results from a blockade of glucose utilization, one might conclude that a primary site of action is at the cell membrane rather than on the microtubular–microfilamentous system. In certain cells, drug action on the plasma membrane may result in the block of the response to the physiological stimulant, such as that observed with the effect of acetylcholine on the adrenal chromaffin cell. In other systems, membrane effects could cause a blockade of certain transport systems, resulting in metabolic aberrations being produced in the cell.

There is little doubt that colchicine and vinblastine bind to tubular protein *in vitro* (Weisenberg *et al.,* 1968; Olmsted and Borisy, 1973), but, again, their actions are not specific in that they precipitate other proteins as well (Redburn *et al.,* 1972; Wuerker and Kirkpatrick, 1972). Thus any attempt to explain the inconclusive—and sometimes contradictory—data by the concept that hormone secretory mechanisms depend on an intact function of microtubules and microfilaments does not appear justified. It is more likely that these systems function in neuronal tissue for the transport of substances from their site of production in the soma to the more distal parts of the axon, rather than for the transport of secretory granules to the cell surface. Their role in nonneuronal secretory organs still has to be elucidated.

CYTOPLASMIC MOTILITY

Instead of postulating the presence of distinct channels by which the secretory granule is guided to the cell membrane, a perhaps more appealing—but still quite speculative—possibility is that the granules are propelled by protoplasmic movement. This would involve either rotational or circulatory movements allowing the granules to move along microstreams. Jahn and Bovee (1969) have developed a general concept of a basic mechanochemical system by which all protoplasms move, which includes muscle contraction and ciliary and flagellar movements, and could even be extended to include secretory phenomena. Motility is presumed to involve the splitting of the high-energy phosphate bonds of ATP by an actomyosin-like protein, and contractile proteins having the same characteristics as muscle actomyosin have been isolated from diverse cell types such as the slime mold, sea urchin eggs, and fibroblasts. The splitting of ATP would provide the energy for the conformational change of the myosin cross-bridge that allows the actin and myosin filaments to slide by each other in a way akin to that proposed for the sliding-filament model of muscle contraction.

Since there is little doubt that ATPase activities have been related to contractile proteins and may be associated with cell motility, it is of interest that ATPase activity is a well-established finding in secretory tissues and inhibition of enzyme activity obtunds the ability of ATP to augment release of secretory product from isolated granule preparations *in vitro* (cf. Rubin, 1970). However, evidence for the existence of contractile actomyosin-like proteins in secretory tissues is not yet well defined. An actomyosin-like protein has been isolated from blood platelets (Lüscher *et al.*, 1972), but its function appears to be involved mainly with platelet aggregation, although a role in the secretory process has not been excluded. An actomyosin-like protein has also been isolated from brain and has been used by its discoverers to support the hypothesis that exocytosis is in part attributable to the chemomechanical action of this actomyosin-like protein (Berl *et al.*, 1973). The isolation of contractile proteins from a variety of other secretory tissues is certainly needed to make this possibility more viable.

The importance of some contractile mechanism in the extrusion process is emphasized by the striking parallelisms between the processes regulating secretion and those regulating contraction, which have previously been considered (cf. Poisner, 1970; Rubin, 1970). The common denominator in secretion and contraction appears to be a transient intracellular accumulation or translocation of calcium ions. The properties of both calcium-dependent activation mechanisms are quite similar, in that, of all other cations tested, only strontium and barium are able to stimulate directly both processes; magnesium and sodium, on the other hand, inhibit the action of calcium in both systems. Further analogies can be made with regard to the metabolic events involved in these two processes. Contraction, like secretion, requires both ATP and calcium ions, and splitting of ATP by ATPase is required in both processes. Thus the most valid conclusion which emerges is that a similar mechanism may exist for triggering these two processes which involves the interaction of calcium, ATP, and ATPase. The action of calcium may be to alter the viscosity of the cytoplasm to facilitate the interaction of the granule membrane with the plasma membrane, or calcium may cooperate with adenine nucleotide in helping to form the connecting link between the two membranes.

If one is willing to accept the close analogy between "stimulus–secretion coupling" and "excitation–contraction coupling," then one must also consider the possibility that calcium regulates secretion through a troponin–tropomyosin-like system. In muscle, troponin and tropomyosin are considered regulatory proteins, in contrast to actin and myosin, which are contractile proteins (Ebashi and Endo, 1968; Ebashi, 1972). Troponin, which is bound to the actin filaments, is thought to be the calcium-receptive protein, and tropomyosin mediates the effect of calcium. In the absence of calcium, troponin, in the presence of tropomyosin, exerts an inhibitory effect on actin filaments. When calcium ions are bound to troponin, this inhibitory action does not take place and contraction follows. Thus, in essence, troponin exerts an inhibitory effect on the interaction of actin and myosin, and calcium ions remove this repression by action on troponin through tropomyosin. The troponin–tropomyosin system is considered here because the hypothesis that calcium initiates contraction by removing an existing repression, rather than by a direct activation, may also provide an explanation for the effects of this cation on secretion. However, experimental validation of this theory requires the isolation of the troponin–tropomyosin system from secretory tissues.

CONCLUSIONS

It is apparent that it is not possible to provide a simple explanation for the nature of calcium's action in modulating the secretory process, and any further speculation concerning the possible mechanism of calcium action on the secretory process at our present state of scientific knowledge would not be fruitful. Although exocytosis appears to be the secretory mechanism in such organs as the adrenal medulla, adrenergic nerve, and neurohypophysis, this process has by no means been proven to exist in all secretory tissues; and indeed in certain organs, such as the thyroid and adrenal cortex, where there is evidence to suggest that secretion may occur by a somewhat different mechanism, the role of calcium in the regulation of secretion has not been clearly defined.

Moreover, in peripheral adrenergic organs the amine releasing activity of tyramine—in contrast to release induced by electric currents—does not seem to occur by exocytosis and does not require the presence of calcium. These observations are compatible with the hypothesis that the role of calcium is related to a fundamental effect on the process of exocytosis, but they do not preclude the possibility that calcium does not have a single action on the secretory mechanism but that its action varies, depending on the mode of secretion of a given organ. There seems little hope of resolving this dilemma until the mechanism of secretion is convincingly ascertained in a wide variety of tissues.

CHAPTER 4

Role of Cyclic AMP in the Secretory Process

The three previous chapters have been devoted to an analysis of the role of calcium in the secretory mechanism, and in order not to obscure the picture which was developed a concerted attempt was made to avoid considering the role of another proposed mediator of the secretory process, adenosine cyclic 3'5'-monophosphate (cyclic AMP). This cyclic nucleotide was isolated by Rall *et al.* (1957) from liver homogenates in the late 1950s during an investigation into the hyperglycemic action of epinephrine. They observed in this cell-free system that cyclic AMP, like epinephrine, is capable of activating liver phosphorylase, and this finding led to the important discovery that the glycogenolytic effect of epinephrine is mediated by cyclic AMP.

Since that original study, a massive amount of evidence has accrued which indicates that the actions of many hormones are mediated through mechanisms involving cyclic AMP; and Sutherland and his many collaborators have put forward the messenger concept to explain the *modus operandi* of cyclic AMP (cf. Robison *et al.*, 1971). This theory affirms that the primary stimulus (first messenger) interacts with sites on the cell membrane to activate adenylate cyclase and produces an increase in cellular cyclic AMP (second messenger). The increase in cyclic AMP leads to an activation of tissue protein kinase, culminating in the physiological response.

The relevance of this model to our present discussion concerns existing evidence implicating cyclic AMP in the regulation of secretory activity which began to appear about the same time Douglas and his associates first elaborated the stimulus–secretion coupling model of secretion. Although the significance of the possible interaction between cyclic AMP and calcium was not immediately realized, it is now well understood by investigators working in this important area of research that elucidating the nature of calcium action on the secretory process requires intimate knowledge of the role of cyclic AMP.

Since Sutherland and his colleagues have laid down certain criteria which they aver, if satisfied, establish that cyclic AMP is an intermediate in hormone action, let us now consider these criteria in relation to the evidence which exists regarding the putative role of cyclic AMP in the secretory mechanism and its interplay with calcium. Our survey and analysis cannot hope to encompass all of the existing evidence in every calcium-dependent secretory system; however, the author has attempted to extract meaningful and informative data from a wide variety of secretory tissues in order to present a coherent picture and ultimately to define in more precise terms the functions of cyclic AMP and calcium in the secretory process.

EFFECTS OF EXOGENOUS CYCLIC NUCLEOTIDE

The first criterion which will be considered involves whether the administration of exogenous cyclic AMP can mimic the effects of the primary secretogogue; i.e., can cyclic AMP directly activate the secretory process? There is little doubt that exogenous administration of cyclic nucleotide to *in vitro* systems can mimic the actions of the trophic hormone on many secretory systems. However, in most tissues the use of the dibutyryl analogue of cyclic AMP is required to produce consistent and dose-related effects. The assumption is that the dibutyryl derivative, being more lipid soluble, is able to penetrate cell membranes more readily and, in addition, is more resistant to the catabolic effects of phosphodies-terase, the enzyme system responsible for the degradation of cyclic AMP (Robison *et al.*, 1971). However, even with the more potent dibutyryl cyclic AMP, millimole concentrations and prolonged exposure times may be required to elicit responses (see, for example, Ridderstap and Bonting, 1969; Nagasawa and Yanai, 1972).

A great deal of study has been carried out on the adenohypophysis, where cyclic AMP or dibutyryl cyclic AMP augments the release of pituitary hormones both *in vitro* and *in vivo*. Thus cyclic nucleotide increases the release of growth hormone (Lockhart Ewart and Taylor, 1971), thyrotropin (Bowers, 1971), adrenocorticotropin (Fleischer *et al.*, 1969; Hedge, 1971), prolactin (Nagasawa and Yanai, 1972), and luteinizing hormone (Zor *et al.*, 1970). The studies *in vitro* indicate that cyclic AMP acts primarily on the release process, rather than on synthesis, since the stimulant effect of cyclic nucleotide is not depressed by inhibitors of protein synthesis and is not associated with any significant effect on incorporation of radioactive amino acid into hormonal polypeptide (Lockhart Ewart and Taylor, 1971; Nagasawa and Yanai, 1972). The response to cyclic AMP, like most other secretogogues, requires the presence of calcium and a source of metabolic energy (Dumont *et al.*, 1971; Lockhart Ewart and Taylor, 1971). Morphological changes in the adenohypophysis were studied by Pelletier *et al.* (1972) after exposure to monobutyryl cyclic AMP, and exocytosis was reported to occur within 5 min after its administration; these investigators feel that such changes are similar to those observed after the injection of hypothalamic hormones *in vivo*. Despite the plethora of data demonstrating the stimulant activity of exogenous cyclic nucleotide on the adenohypophysis, the author is not aware of any existing evidence which shows that cyclic AMP is able to elicit similar effects on the neurohypophysis.

Exogenous cyclic nucleotide is also able to trigger the release of insulin from isolated pancreatic islets (Malaisse *et al.*, 1967), from the isolated perfused pancreas (Basabe *et al.*, 1971), and from perfused rat islets (Charles *et al.*, 1973). In the perfused rat islet preparations the effect of cyclic AMP is very rapid, with a twofold increase in insulin secretion occurring within 2 min (Charles *et al.*, 1973). Cyclic nucleotide is also able to augment steroidogenesis in a variety of *in vitro* adrenal preparations (Robison *et al.*, 1971), but its effect on catecholamine release from intact adrenal glands has generally been inconsequential (Smith and Winkler, 1972), although there has been one positive report of an enhancement of catecholamine secretion after the injection of dibutyryl cyclic AMP into the cat adrenal gland perfused retrograde (Peach, 1972).

The finding that exogenous cyclic nucleotide can induce thyrocalcitonin release is of special interest, since the secretion of this hormone appears to be regulated directly by calcium, with no prior stimulation needed to activate or translocate calcium. The effect of cyclic nucleotide is demonstrable *in situ* (Avioli *et al.*, 1971; Care *et al.*, 1971a), although much higher concentrations are required to stimulate calcitonin secretion by thyroid slices (Bell, 1970). The ability of cyclic AMP to induce calcitonin release—which is directly monitored by calcium without the intervention of any other stimulating agent—would imply that any potential role of cyclic AMP in hormone release is related to some calcium-mediated effect on the secretory process and not to some ancillary effect on the primary stimulating agent.

However, the interrelation between calcium and cyclic AMP is made more complex when it is revealed that cyclic AMP can also induce the release of parathyroid hormone (Williams *et al.*, 1973). Any universal concept of a calcium–cyclic AMP synergism to induce release is made less viable when it is recalled that although calcium regulates parathyroid hormone secretion, the relationship is an inverse one; in this system, calcium acts like magnesium to inhibit hormone release (Sherwood *et al.*, 1970). The possibility has been considered that calcium may regulate parathyroid hormone secretion by an action on synthesis, and the antagonistic effects of cyclic AMP on calcium action may thus occur at the level of hormone biosynthesis—although there is no direct evidence to support such a hypothesis.

The stimulant action of pituitary thyrotropin on the thyroid gland is associated not only with an increase in turnover and release of thyroid hormone but also with certain metabolic changes, such as an increase in glucose oxidation and in phospholipid turnover (Dumont *et al.*, 1971). The effect of dibutyryl cyclic AMP has been reported to reproduce faithfully all of the effects of thyrotropin (Ahn and Rosenberg, 1970; Knopp *et al.*, 1970). Thus in certain *in vitro* systems dibutyryl cyclic AMP can cause an increase in glucose oxidation, in phospholipid turnover, and in the formation of colloid droplets; in the absence of calcium, the stimulation of glucose oxidation is markedly reduced, whereas colloid endocytosis or thyroid secretion is not significantly affected (Zor *et al.*, 1968; Dumont *et al.*, 1971). These studies have been used to support the notion that cyclic AMP mimics the actions of pituitary thyrotropin.

However, conflicting evidence dictates circumspection before accepting this perhaps too simplistic conclusion. In most of these studies, cyclic AMP has little or no stimulant actions, although its dibutyryl derivative is much more active. It has been assumed that the increased potency of dibutyryl cyclic AMP over cyclic AMP is merely due to its more nonpolar nature, which makes it easier to penetrate cell membranes. However, there is really no direct evidence that dibutyryl cyclic AMP is merely an innocuous substitute for cyclic AMP, and indeed it does not always mimic the actions of cyclic AMP. Although many of the actions of dibutyryl cyclic AMP on the thyroid gland are similar to those of thyrotropin, Pastan and Macchia (1967) have shown species differences in the metabolic responses *in vitro* to this cyclic AMP analogue, and these two cyclic analogues have divergent effects on both iodide trapping and ^{14}C transport (Burke *et al.*, 1971). Moreover, in isolated fat cells cyclic AMP increases the production of carbon dioxide and lipogenesis, whereas the dibutyryl analogue inhibits this conversion. In Hela cells, dibutyryl cyclic AMP decreases the glycogen content, whereas cyclic AMP increases the glycogen content (see Burke *et al.*, 1971). Such findings emphasize that caution should be employed in drawing conclusions of physiological mechanisms from effects produced by pharmacological concentrations of a chemical analogue whose mechanism of action is still in doubt.

Dibutyryl cyclic AMP can also increase salivary secretion from the rat parotid *in vitro*, as first demonstrated by Schramm and his coworkers (Babad *et al.*, 1967). Although dibutyryl cyclic AMP may be as effective as epinephrine in inducing enzyme secretion and requires the presence of calcium (Selinger and Naim, 1970), the finding that epinephrine-induced potassium release and vacuole formation cannot be reproduced by cyclic nucleotide indicates that cyclic AMP is not an essential intermediate in all of the manifestations of catecholamine action (Batzri *et al.*, 1971). In the insect salivary gland, exogenous cyclic AMP also does not mimic the effects of the primary hormone, 5-hydroxytryptamine (serotonin), in that cyclic AMP induces hyperpolarization of the membrane, whereas 5-hydroxytryptamine causes depolarization (Berridge and Prince, 1972).

In view of the morphological and functional resemblance between the parotid gland and exocrine pancreas, one might expect that cyclic AMP enhances exocrine secretion from the pancreas; but the evidence which presently exists in this regard is conflicting. However, in certain *in vitro* systems, exposure to millimolar concentrations of cyclic AMP for an hour or more can lead to enhanced secretion of pancreatic amylase (Ridderstap and Bonting, 1969; Bauduin *et al.*, 1971). Although the activity of dibutyryl cyclic AMP as a pancreatic secretogogue is obtunded by calcium deprivation, Heisler *et al.*, (1972) find that whereas manganese inhibits the secretory response to carbachol it does not affect the secretory response to exogenous cyclic nucleotide. This significant finding suggests that cyclic AMP does not cause a transmembrane movement of calcium and that the critical calcium fraction utilized by exogenous cyclic nucleotide is different from the fraction utilized in cholinergic stimulation. In accord with this conclusion is the inability of cyclic nucleotide to affect the membrane potential of pancreatic acinar cells (Matthews and Petersen, 1973).

Although the stimulatory effect of cyclic AMP is usually discernible in tissue slices and in other types of *in vitro* systems, this cyclic nucleotide, or its dibutyryl analogue, is much less effective in intact tissues. For example, Morisset and Webster (1971) found that the administration of dibutyryl cyclic AMP to the intact rat was associated with an initial decrease followed by a slight increase in amylase secretion, whereas cyclic AMP was able to augment amylase secretion *in vitro*, although prolonged exposure (1 hr) was needed. In a similar vein, dibutyryl cyclic AMP increases water and electrolyte but not amylase secretion from the intact perfused cat pancreas (Case and Scratcherd, 1972a). Case and Scratcherd conclude from these latter results that dibutyryl cyclic AMP is able to mimic the physiological actions of secretin on water and electrolyte secretion, but it does not mimic the actions of pancreozymin on protein secretion.

Evidence demonstrating that exogenous cyclic nucleotide can induce neurotransmitter release is not at all convincing. Goldberg and Singer (1969) reported that dibutyryl cyclic AMP in the rather high concentration of 4 mM increases the amplitude of the end-plate potential in isolated rat diaphragm and increases the frequency but not amplitude of the spontaneous miniature end-plate potentials. These findings may be expected if the cyclic nucleotide increases the release of transmitter packets of acetylcholine. Goldberg and Singer suggested that cyclic AMP may promote glycolytic metabolism in nerve endings, which in turn modulates rate of release. However, Ginsborg and Hirst (1972) subsequently uncovered findings in conflict with this notion. They found that adenosine, which increases cyclic AMP levels in brain, decreases the quantum content of end-plate potentials, and they conclude that if cyclic AMP is directly involved in neurotransmitter release it is probably to decrease rather than promote release.

Adrenergic nerves also appear to respond to high concentrations of cyclic nucleotide. Dibutyryl cyclic AMP enhances norepinephrine and dopamine β-hydroxylase release from the guinea pig vas deferens induced by nerve stimulation, and dibutyryl cyclic AMP also increases spontaneous release (Wooten *et al.*, 1973). The stimulant effect of cyclic nucleotide is profoundly reduced by calcium deprivation. Although cyclic nucleotide can apparently elicit catecholamine release from peripheral adrenergic nerves, it has generally been ineffective as an adrenomedullary secretogogue, although Peach (1972) found that bolus injections of cyclic AMP or its dibutyryl derivative increase catecholamine secretion from the cat adrenal gland perfused retrograde; he further observed that perfusion with calcium-free solution had no detrimental effect on cyclic AMP–induced release. It is of interest that prolonged perfusion of cat adrenal glands via the arterial circulation with high concentrations of cyclic AMP or dibutyryl cyclic AMP does not elicit augmented rates of release (Jaanus and Rubin, unpublished observations). The reason for this discrepancy between the effects of cyclic nucleotide on glands perfused retrograde and *in situ* is unclear.

Up to now, we have considered only the facilitatory activity of cyclic AMP as a secretogogue, but in certain calcium-dependent secretory systems it appears that it is also able to act as an inhibitor of the secretory process. The inhibitory action of cyclic AMP has been demonstrated with histamine release by anaphylaxis (Lichtenstein, 1971) and 48/80 (Loeffler *et al.*, 1971) and with the thrombin-induced platelet release reaction (Salzman *et al.*, 1972). This evidence is of a circumstantial nature, since high concentrations of dibutyryl cyclic AMP are required, but is nevertheless compatible with the hypothesis that cyclic AMP, rather than being an inducer of release, can protect the cell against the extrusion of product. Possible sites at which cyclic AMP can exert its inhibitory effects are at the level of the cell membrane or in the energy-requiring process concerned with granule expulsion. Although a choice between these two alternatives is still a matter of conjecture, some insight into the nature of the effect may be found in the fact that inhibition by dibutyryl cyclic AMP of histamine release occurs primarily in an early stage of the release process, so that—whether it is a physiological phenomenon or not—the effect of exogenous cyclic nucleotide appears to be at the level of the cell membrane.

We have seen that the release of gastric juice involves a calcium-dependent process, and Harris and his collaborators (Harris and Alonso, 1965) developed the hypothesis that cyclic AMP acts as a "second messenger" between secretogogues and chemical reactions involved in active transport of hydrochloric acid by the stomach. Among the pieces of evidence they uncovered was that exogenous cyclic AMP was able to augment acid secretion from the amphibian gastric mucosa. On the other hand, in man and dog there is no evidence for the role of cyclic AMP in acid secretion, and, in fact, a cyclic AMP infusion may inhibit secretion in response to histamine or gastrin (Levine and Wilson, 1971; Mao *et al.*, 1972).

The variable effects of cyclic AMP on acid secretion could be explained on the basis of species variability, which does not provide much comfort to those interested in developing universal theories. Alternatively, the effects of exogenous cyclic nucleotide on gastric secretion may be related to alterations in blood flow However, since cyclic AMP–induced gastric acid secretion is associated with increased oxygen consumption and glycogenolysis, it is not clear whether the secretory response to cyclic AMP, when present, is a consequence of direct effects on hydrogen ion transport or is related to an effect on intermediary metabolism.

It is clear from the evidence presented that in most *in vitro* systems cyclic AMP can augment the release reaction. The large concentrations required to induce secretion in intact tissues may be explained on the basis of permeability factors, and one can point to the fact that the more lipid-soluble dibutyryl analogue of cyclic AMP is generally a more potent secretogogue. This is certainly a valid argument, as exemplified by the author's own experience; for whereas cyclic nucleotides have no effect on steroid production or release from the intact perfused cat adrenal gland (Carchman *et al.*, 1971; Rubin *et al.*, 1972), cyclic AMP enhances steroid production in these same cat adrenocortical cells when they are studied in isolation after trypsin digestion (Warner and Rubin, unpublished observations). Furthermore, there is no doubt that any *in vivo* study of the effects of cyclic nucleotide, or any other secretogogue, is made difficult by the many neural and humoral factors which may influence the secretory response. Although many of these factors can be controlled *in vitro*, such investigations are hindered by problems of diffusion of substances into and out of tissues, as well as by excessive spontaneous release which may mask the stimulant activity of the secretogogue. There are therefore a number of valid explanations to account for weak activity of exogenous cyclic nucleotide, when it is found.

On the other hand, there are other reasons to question whether high concentrations of cyclic nucleotide administered to isolated systems can be considered as representing a duplication of the events occurring in the intact tissue under physiological conditions. Nucleotides in high concentrations can be toxic to cells (Robison *et al.*, 1971), and toxic substances will induce the release response from a variety of tissues, presumably through nonphysiological mechanisms. Furthermore, if administered cyclic AMP is acting as a "second messenger" and mimics the effect of the primary hormone, then it should manifest a similar dependence on calcium; but this clearly is not the case. The reader should consult the studies of Peach (1972) on the perfused cat adrenal gland, Haksar and Peron (1972) on adrenocortical tissue *in vitro*, Heisler *et al.* (1972) on the exocrine pancreas, and Malaisse and coworkers (Brisson *et al.*, 1972) on the endocrine pancreas, which all illustrate the very critical point that although the secretory activity of exogenous cyclic nucleotide may be facilitated by calcium, the calcium pool mobilized by exogenous cyclic AMP or its dibutyryl derivative is not the same as that mobilized by the trophic hormone. This makes it highly unlikely that administered cyclic nucleotide is evoking release through a mechanism identical to the physiological stimulus. This idea is supported by data obtained from studies on other secretory tissues, such as the thyroid (Burke *et al.*, 1971) and salivary glands (Batzri *et al.*, 1971), which unequivocally demonstrate that the metabolic and morphological activities associated with the secretory response to cyclic AMP are not identical to those observed with the primary stimulus.

PHOSPHODIESTERASE INHIBITION

If the addition of exogenous cyclic nucleotide to secretory tissues does not represent a completely satisfactory way to elucidate its physiological role in the release process, then another approach would be to augment the levels of endogenous cyclic nucleotide by inhibiting its degradation. The catabolism of cyclic AMP is catalyzed by specific phosphodiesterases which are located in multiple molecular forms primarily in the cytoplasm. By rapidly hydrolyzing cyclic AMP to 5'-AMP, the diesterases prevent its accumulation and thereby play a key role in terminating its action. A number of pharmacological agents, most notably the methylxanthines and the opiate alkaloid, papaverine, inhibit this enzyme system and allow cyclic AMP to increase in the cell. Theophylline has proven to be a particularly useful methylxanthine in this regard, although caffeine has also been commonly employed.

Papaverine, while a more potent inhibitor of phosphodiesterase, has to be used with caution, since it may influence secretory rates by its activity as a vascular smooth muscle relaxant and a metabolic poison.

In some secretory systems, methylxanthines—generally in high concentrations—will augment the basal rate of release from the adenohypophysis both *in vitro* (Fleischer *et al.*, 1969; Kudo *et al.*, 1972) and *in vivo* (Hedge, 1971); from the exocrine (Heisler *et al.*, 1972) and endocrine pancreas (Charles *et al.*, 1973); from the salivary gland (Kulka and Sternlicht, 1968); from the parathyroid gland (Williams *et al.*, 1973); from the thyroid gland [thyroid hormone (Dumont *et al.*, 1971) and calcitonin (Avioli *et al.*, 1971)]; from the adrenal medula (Poisner, 1973); and from adrenergic (Wooten *et al.*, 1973) and cholinergic nerves (Goldberg and Singer, 1969). In other systems, phosphodiesterase inhibitors do not by themselves augment release but do potentiate the secretory responses to other secretogogues, as well as to exogenous cyclic nucleotide. This appears to be the case for certain pancreas preparations, where methylxanthine may not affect insulin release from pancreatic islets *in vitro* in the absence of glucose but markedly enhances glucose-induced insulin release at high glucose concentrations (Lambert *et al.*, 1969b; Brisson *et al.*, 1972). Such findings might suggest that theophylline acts by somehow facilitating glucose metabolism in the β cell; however, theophylline enhances the secretory response to amino acids—in the absence of glucose (Milner, 1970)—so the effect of theophylline and that of cyclic AMP are not specifically directed on glucose metabolism; however, this finding does not rule out the possibility that cyclic AMP can indirectly influence secretion by effects on other metabolic phenomena occurring in β cells—or any other secretory cell, for that matter.

Methylxanthines also potentiate the secretory response to exogenous cyclic nucleotide (Bell, 1970; Bauduin *et al.*, 1971), although in certain systems, such as the exocrine pancreas, the facilitatory effect of theophylline is not extended to physiological stimuli such as pancreozymin and cholinergic agents (Bauduin *et al.*, 1971; Heisler *et al.*, 1972). These data raise doubt as to whether the secretory response to exogenous cyclic nucleotide and/or theophylline is mediated through the same mechanism as the primary physiological stimulus. This point attains added validity when one becomes cognizant of the fact that while diazoxide—a chemical analogue of the thiazide diuretics—inhibits the enhanced secretion of insulin induced by glucose, it has no effect on insulin release produced by theophylline or cyclic AMP (Basabe *et al.*, 1971).

The trend of the data presented so far indicates that cyclic AMP is not a rate-limiting factor in the secretory response, although it may play an ancillary or indirect role in this process. Rasmussen (1970) first proposed that cyclic AMP modulates the secretory process by an effect on calcium metabolism, and so agents which inhibit phosphodiesterase might increase cell calcium levels by increasing tissue cyclic AMP. However, there is little direct evidence in support of this hypothesis. The stimulant effect of theophylline and caffeine is probably the result of a *direct* mobilization of calcium, analogous to their actions on intracellular calcium pools in muscle. Bianchi (1968) originally suggested that these agents reduce calcium binding to intracellular components such as the sarcoplasmic reticulum in muscle and through this mechanism produce an increase in intracellular ionized calcium.

It is of interest that the secretory responses to methylxanthines, like the secretory response to exogenous cyclic nucleotide, appear to be less dependent on the presence of extracellular calcium than the physiological stimulus. This phenomenon has been observed with insulin release from the pancreas (Brisson *et al.*, 1972) and with catecholamine release from both the adrenal medulla (Poisner, 1973) and sympathetic nerves (Wooten *et al.*, 1973). There is reason to believe that this disparity is attributable to the fact that an intracellular calcium pool is critical for xanthine-induced secretion, which is distinct from the extracellular calcium fraction required, for example, to sustain acetylcholine-mediated catecholamine secretion or glucose-induced insulin release.

Kinetic studies show that whereas glucose increases radiocalcium uptake and decreases efflux from isolated pancreatic islet cells, theophylline and cyclic AMP have variable effects on calcium uptake and enhance efflux (Brisson *et al.*, 1972). This is convincing evidence that in the very few instances where effects on calcium metabolism can be demonstrated by theophylline and cyclic AMP, they do not resemble those of the primary physiological stimulus and therefore point to a different mechanism of action. But whether or not theophylline exerts its actions primarily by modulating calcium metabolism, it may very well act through some cyclic AMP–dependent mechanism, since the effects of cyclic AMP or dibutyryl cyclic AMP on release are more readily potentiated by the methylxanthines than the effects of the primary stimulating agent. There is no doubt that theophylline can increase tissue cyclic AMP levels in such secretory tissues as the adrenal cortex (Carchman *et al.*, 1971), adenohypophysis (Steiner *et al.*, 1970), and exocrine (Benz *et al.*, 1972) and endocrine pancreas (Charles *et al.*, 1973), but it is still unclear whether the facilitatory effect of theophylline and other inhibitors of phosphodiesterase on the secretory process is primarily the result of this action.

MEASUREMENT OF CYCLIC AMP LEVELS

The relative nonspecificity of action of most pharmacologically active substances requires us to question whether the observed responses to high concentrations of cyclic nucleotide and methylxanthine are really the direct result of their anticipated effects; this tends to mitigate the significance of such data in elucidating the physiological role of cyclic AMP. Since cyclic AMP is widely distributed in secretory organs, another approach employed involves a study of the relationship between tissue cyclic AMP levels and the secretory response. If cyclic AMP exerts direct control over the rate of secretion, then an enhanced secretory response might be expected to be accompanied by an increase in cyclic AMP; conversely, an increase in the concentration of cyclic AMP should augment the secretory rate. Let us therefore examine what is known of the changes which occur in the levels of cyclic AMP during activation of the secretory mechanism.

It is generally conceded that exposure of a variety of secretory tissues to physiological stimuli is usually associated with activation of adenylate cyclase and an increase in cyclic AMP (Robison *et al.*, 1971). The following secretory tissues manifest such an increase following stimulation: the pancreas with secretin or pancreozymin

(Benz *et al.*, 1972), adrenal cortex with ACTH (Grahame-Smith *et al.*, 1967), adenohypophysis with hypothalamic extract (Zor *et al.*, 1970; Borgeat *et al.*, 1972), thyroid gland with TSH (Gilman and Rall, 1968; Knopp *et al.*, 1970), and gastric tissue with histamine and pentagastrin (Bieck, 1972). In certain tissues, such as the adrenal cortex (Carchman *et al.*, 1971), adenohypophysis (Bowers, 1971), and stomach (Bieck, 1972), stimulation may also be associated with an increase in cyclic AMP in the perfusate or incubation medium; moreover, in the stomach the augmented cyclic AMP secretion triggered by histamine or pentagastrin precedes maximum acid secretion. The increase in tissue cyclic AMP levels also generally precedes the augmented secretory response. This has been clearly shown in the responses to ACTH in the perfused cat adrenal gland (Carchman. *et al.*, 1971), to secretin in the perfused cat pancreas (Case *et al.*, 1972), and to hypothalamic thyrotropin releasing factor in the rat pituitary *in vitro* (Bowers, 1971).

The inability to detect any changes in tissue cyclic AMP during stimulation could be explained by a number of possibilities. It is conceivable that the increase in cyclic AMP is very transient and is therefore not easily detectable with techniques currently available. Alternatively, the heterogeneity of a given tissue may make it difficult to detect small changes in the cyclic AMP concentrations, especially if these small changes are limited to a

Although a quantitative correlation between the ability of a given secretogogue to augment cyclic AMP levels and to elicit the physiological response has been demonstrated in a few secretory systems, in others relatively low concentrations of the physiological stimulus evoke a release response in the absence of any detectable increase in cyclic AMP concentrations. Montague and Cook (1971) found that glucose (5–20 mM) increases insulin secretion from isolated pancreatic islet cells without any measurable increase in tissue cyclic AMP. Pancreozymin and secretin augment amylase release from rat pancreas *in vitro*, with no effect on cyclic AMP levels (Benz *et al.*, 1972), and low doses of ACTH augment steroid production in isolated rat adrenal cells, with no measurable increase in cyclic AMP (Beall and Sayers, 1972) (Fig. 19).

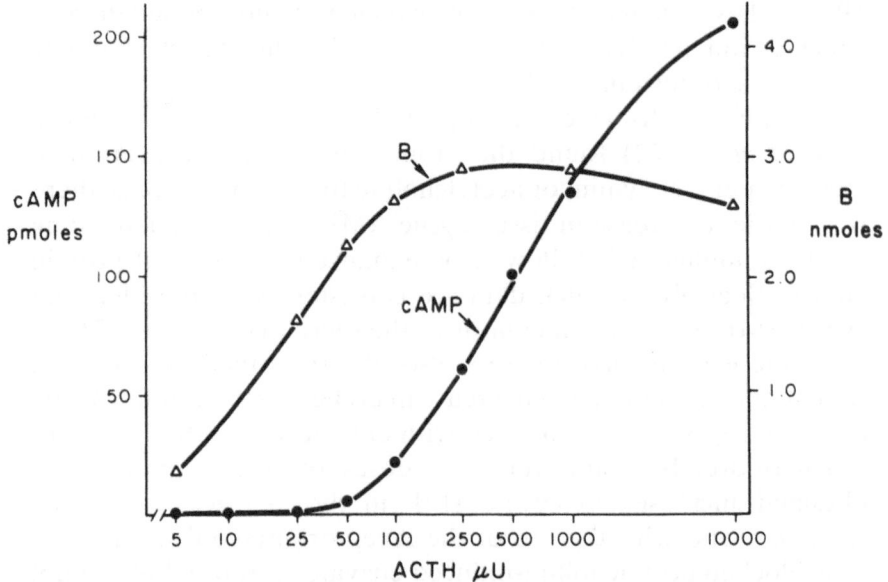

Fig. 19. Accumulation of cyclic AMP (CAMP) and of corticosterone (B) after addition of ACTH to isolated rat adrenocortical cells (Beall and Sayers, 1972).

cell compartment which represents a minute fraction of the tissue under study. However, the inability to detect augmented cyclic AMP concentrations in the relatively homogeneous isolated rat adrenocortical cell preparation with low ACTH concentrations makes this last presumption somewhat more difficult to accept (Fig. 19).

Since investigations up to now have not resolved whether increased cyclic AMP levels are a *sine qua non* for activation of the secretory mechanism, an alternate approach to this problem is to examine whether increases in cyclic AMP concentrations are consistently related to an enhanced secretory response; and this appears not to be the case. In the pancreas, for example, inhibition of phosphodiesterase is associated with marked increases in cyclic AMP levels but little or no enhancement of insulin release (Montague and Cook, 1971; Charles *et al.*, 1973). The presence of glucose is required for the induction of insulin secretion, and these secretory events are not necessarily accompanied by significant changes in cyclic AMP concentrations (Montague and Cook,

1971). These results, obtained by two separate groups, led them to conclude independently that cyclic AMP does not directly mediate the release of insulin.

Similar results have been reported in other secretory systems. Case *et al.* (1972) found that, following the administration of secretin, pancreozymin, or acetylcholine to the cat pancreas, there is a transient increase in tissue cyclic AMP levels, and, depending on the stimulus, it is followed by enhanced secretion of protein and/or electrolytes. Such data are consistent with the idea that cyclic AMP is a direct mediator of the secretory response. However, these same investigators also observed that, as secretion waned, the accompanying decrease in cyclic AMP was followed by a secondary rise not associated with enhanced secretin (Fig. 20). Furthermore, by using very low doses of pancreozymin they obtained increases in cyclic AMP in the absence of enzyme secretion, and with the use of the receptor antagonist, atropine, they blocked acetylcholine-induced enzyme secretion but did not

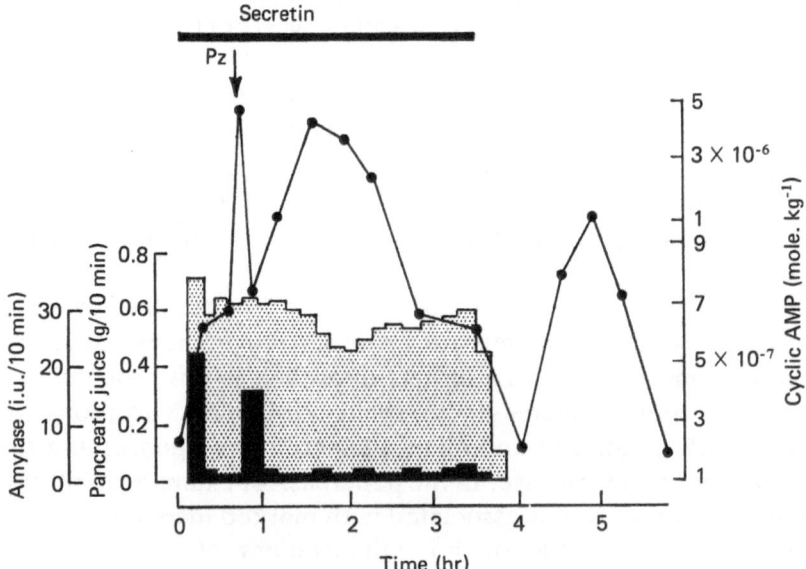

Fig. 20. Effect of an intravenous injection of pancreozymin (5 mg) on pancreatic amylase secretion (black bars) and on the concentration of cyclic AMP (black dots) in the cat pancreas during submaximal electrolyte secretion (stippled bars) in response to an infusion of secretin (Case *et al.*, 1972).

affect the concomitant rise in cyclic AMP concentration. Case and his colleagues concluded from this study that while one could not rule out that cyclic AMP is necessary for secretion of electrolytes and enzymes, secretion does not necessarily follow an increase in cyclic AMP concentrations.

Bowers and his collaborators (Bowers, 1971) observed similar phenomena when they attempted to correlate cyclic AMP levels and thyrotropin secretion *in vitro* from the rat pituitary gland. Theophylline, while increasing cyclic AMP, elicited no increase in thyrotropin release. Moreover, at a time when cyclic AMP concentrations were at maximum levels as the result of prolonged exposure to hypothalamic releasing factor, hormone release was at its nadir. Such studies are compatible with our own findings that cation deprivation will cause marked increases in cyclic AMP in adrenal gland and perfusate, although no increase in corticosteroid release is demonstrable unless ACTH is also present (Carchman *et al.*, 1971). The trend of the various findings thus indicates that activation of the secretory mechanism can clearly be dissociated from increased tissue levels of cyclic AMP; it further suggests that the physiological stimulus is triggering the release reaction by an effect not directly mediated by changes in tissue cyclic AMP.

Although a close functional relationship between cyclic AMP and hormone release has not been established, cyclic AMP appears to be involved in hormone synthesis. Our own studies have clearly shown that although an increase in adrenal cyclic AMP levels is not sufficient to trigger corticosteroid release, this increase in cyclic AMP is associated with enhanced steroid synthesis and turnover provided calcium is present (Rubin *et al.*, 1972). This apparent association between tissue cyclic AMP levels and hormone synthesis has also been extended to the adrenal medulla, where Guidotti and Costa (1973) have found that changes in medullary cyclic AMP are more closely related to induction of tyrosine hydroxylase—the rate-limiting enzyme for catecholamine synthesis—than to catecholamine release. However, further studies on intact secretory systems are needed to establish more definitively whether the action of cyclic AMP is universally on synthesis.

INTERACTION BETWEEN CALCIUM
AND CYCLIC AMP

Although it is not possible to establish a correlation between cyclic AMP levels and secretory rate, it should be realized that the action of cyclic AMP may be effected through another mediator. The idea that cyclic AMP might activate the secretory process by enhancing the mobilization of calcium is an attractive possibility and must be given consideration; it gains credence when one recalls that while calcium is required for expression of the effects of cyclic AMP, it is not required for cyclic nucleotide synthesis. In the absence of calcium, stimulation is still associated with increases in cyclic AMP in the salivary gland (Rasmussen and Tenenhouse, 1968), thyroid gland (Dekker and Field, 1970), adenohypophysis (Steiner et al., 1970), and adrenal cortex (Carchman et al., 1971).

Since calcium deprivation does not depress cyclic AMP production, the question arises as to whether cyclic AMP modulates calcium metabolism, as, for example, by altering the permeability of cell membranes to calcium. At present there is little or no conclusive evidence which shows that cyclic AMP alters calcium distribution in tissues in a way consistent with the idea that this cyclic nucleotide plays a critical role in stimulus–secretion coupling. Thus we have already alluded to the fact that although dibutyryl cyclic AMP and theophylline do indeed alter the kinetics of calcium flux in the pancreas, these effects are markedly different from those of the physiological stimulus, glucose (Brisson et al., 1972). Alterations in membrane potential are generally considered manifestations of changes in transmembrane ion fluxes, and in the insect salivary gland the physiological mediator, 5-hydroxytryptamine, which can augment cyclic AMP synthesis, produces a calcium-dependent membrane depolarization, whereas exogenous cyclic nucleotide or theophylline produces hyperpolarization (Berridge and Prince, 1972). By inference, it appears that in this system the ion fluxes triggered by cyclic AMP are also different from those triggered by the physiological mediator, and this conclusion has recently been corroborated by direct experimental analysis (Prince et al., 1972).

Additional salient information concerning the direct effects of cyclic AMP on calcium metabolism in other secretory systems is sadly lacking. High concentrations of exogenously administered cyclic AMP increase calcium efflux from the perfused rat liver (Williams *et al.*, 1971). These data, obtained from a tissue whose primary function involves metabolic as well as secretory activity, demonstrate that high concentrations of exogenous cyclic AMP can alter transmembrane calcium movement. Effects of cyclic AMP on isolated membrane system such as the sarcoplasmic reticulum have so far been inconsistent (cf. Entman *et al.*, 1969; Sulakhe and Dhalla, 1970), but if this proves a real phenomenon it could suggest a physiological role for cyclic AMP in the transport of cellular calcium.

If cyclic AMP does not affect calcium metabolism, another possible mode of action may involve the activation of cellular protein. Since the initial report by Krebs and coworkers (Walsh *et al.*, 1968) of a cyclic AMP–dependent protein kinase in skeletal muscle which can stimulate the phosphorylation of a wide spectrum of proteins, a similar enzyme system has been found in liver, brain, and adipose tissue. It has also been identified and characterized in such nonneuronal secretory tissues as the adrenal cortex (Garren *et al.*, 1971), adenohypophysis (Labrie *et al.*, 1971), and endocrine pancreas (Montague and Howell, 1973). Rasmussen and his colleagues (Goodman *et al.*, 1970) have attempted to explain the effects of cyclic AMP on secretion by proposing that it activates the phosphorylation of microtubular protein, which is then followed by calcium activation of the phosphorylated protein. This theory—which implies that the calcium requirement for cyclic AMP–induced release of hormones is not due to a direct stimulant effect of this cation on cyclic AMP–activated protein kinase—derives support from studies on pituitary protein kinase (Labrie *et al.*, 1971).

Gillespie (1971) has also considered the interaction of cyclic AMP and calcium in relation to a microtubular system—but one which is directly involved with cell motility. She proposes that calcium affects cell function and perhaps enhances release by promoting the formation of microtubules from available subunits; low concentrations of cyclic AMP, by mobilizing calcium, would favor microtubule formation, while at higher concentrations the cyclic nucleotide would act in an opposite manner to increase the pool of available subunits.

The most interesting aspect of this speculative theory lies in the fact that, if valid, it would explain some of the existing stimulatory and inhibitory effects of cyclic AMP and calcium on secretion. We have seen that calcium is an inhibitor of parathyroid secretion, whereas exogenous cyclic nucleotide enhances its release. Calcium augments, while cyclic AMP inhibits, histamine release. In other secretory systems, both calcium and cyclic AMP are facilitatory. Thus if cyclic AMP does play a direct role in the secretory mechanism, then a theory such as Gillespie's will be necessary to explain both the facilitatory and the inhibitory actions of cyclic AMP and calcium. Another aspect of this problem which tends to militate against a specific role for cyclic AMP in the release process is that other cyclic nucleotides, such as cyclic GMP (guanosine cyclic 3'5'-monophosphate), are also found in a variety of tissues, and any potential relationship of cyclic AMP to the secretory mechanism must also include one or more of these other cyclic nucleotides.

PROSTAGLANDINS

There exists a family of unsaturated fatty acids called the prostaglandins which, being ubiquitously distributed and having a wide variety of endocrine and metabolic effects (Bergström *et al.*, 1968), have also been implicated as modulators of the release process.

Prostaglandins induce release from various glands (cf. Flack, 1973), including the exocrine (Case and Scratcherd, 1972b) and endocrine pancreas (Bressler *et al.*, 1968), adenohypophysis (MacLeod and Lehmeyer, 1970; Hertelendy, 1971; Hedge, 1972), thyroid (Dekker and Field, 1970), and adrenal cortex (Saruta and Kaplan, 1972). Moreover, certain prostaglandins (E series) are at least as potent or even more potent inducers of corticosteroid production and growth hormone release than cyclic nucleotide or theophylline (Hertelendy, 1971; Flack and Ramwell, 1972). The difficulty in accurately determining precise tissue levels of prostaglandins has impeded investigators from correlating tissue concentrations with the physiological release response. However, an increase in prostaglandin release has been observed after stimulation of the cat adrenal gland, spleen, and stomach (cf. Ramwell and Rabinowitz, 1972). The amount released appears to be much higher than the tissue concentrations, which makes it likely that secretory activity is associated with an increase in prostaglandin synthesis. Although prostaglandin release appears to coincide with the secretory response, the cellular locus of prostglandin synthesis and release cannot be precisely ascertained in these organs, since they are heterogeneous tissues, composed of a variety of cell types.

Investigations concerning the nature of prostaglandin action in the secretory mechanism have raised the possibility that the adenylate cyclase–cyclic AMP system is involved. Prostaglandins stimulate thyroid (Field *et al.*, 1971) and adenohypophyseal adenylate cyclase *in vitro* (Zor *et al.*, 1970), and some correlation has been established between growth hormone (Steiner *et al.*, 1970) and thyroid hormone (Sato *et al.*, 1972) release and tissue levels of cyclic AMP. The secretory activity of prostaglandins bears certain other resemblances to cyclic nucleotide–induced release. Thus their activity depends on the presence of calcium (Hertelendy, 1971; Saruta and Kaplan, 1972) and is potentiated by theophylline (Hertelendy, 1971; Case and Scratcherd, 1972b), and in certain tissues such as the stomach (Shaw and Ramwell, 1968; Way and Durbin, 1969), blood platelets (Mürer, 1971), and adrenergic nerves (Hedqvist, 1970) they inhibit release rather than facilitate it. The inhibitory effect of prostaglandin on the thrombin-induced platelet release reaction is similar to that of cyclic nucleotide, and may even be mediated through cyclic AMP, since prostaglandin augments cyclase activity of blood platelets (Marquis *et al.*, 1969) and increases cyclic AMP levels (Droller and Wolfe, 1972). But, in contrast to the inhibitory effects of exogenously administered prostaglandins on the release response from adrenergic neurons and the stomach, the administration of cyclic AMP to similar test systems may enhance release (Wooten *et al.*, 1973).

It is thus apparent that though prostaglandins have both stimulatory and inhibitory actions in many secretory systems which are similar to those of cyclic AMP, there are also exceptions to this rule. And indeed the proposal has been made that prostaglandins are involved in the secretory process in a different way from cyclic AMP. According to this concept, stimulation brings about prostaglandin release from tissues, which in turn interacts with the adenylate cyclase system to reduce the formation of cyclic AMP and limits hormone action by negative feedback inhibition (Ramwell and Shaw, 1970). An obvious deterrent to accepting this theory is that prostaglandins do not inhibit the secretory response in all instances, but, as pointed out above, like cyclic AMP they are more likely to be facilitatory.

The findings that prostaglandins mimic the effects of cyclic AMP in certain tissues while in other tissues they exert inhibitory effects on certain cyclic AMP–mediated responses may signify that prostaglandins do not act through cyclic AMP but by modifying calcium flux (Ramwell and Shaw, 1970; Ramwell and Rabinowitz, 1972). But there is no direct evidence from secretory tissues in support of this postulate. Critical analysis of the existing data indicates that the primary factor which determines the rate of release is the intracellular accumulation of calcium ions brought about by a direct effect of the *primary stimulus*. Documentation of this concept was provided in Chapter 2 by numerous examples of direct experimental evidence.

It is clear from the foregoing discussion that the role of prostaglandins in the secretory process—like that of cyclic AMP—remains an enigma. Although there has been a plethora of experimentation on the effects of prostaglandins on secretory organs, no physiological function for these substances has been established. Since the doses of prostaglandins required to show effects on secretion are generally much higher than the amounts found in most tissues, it is still unresolved whether these substances do act at a physiologically relevant level to modulate directly the secretory mechanism. They could exert some indirect role by controlling access of the primary secretogogue to secretory cells, as, for example, by acting as a functional vasodilator or vasoconstrictor. But despite the vast amount of recent interest in this area of research, all that can be said at present is that if prostaglandins do directly participate in the secretory process a complex interrelation must exist between these substances and cyclic AMP and calcium.

CONCLUSIONS

Although the translocation of calcium appears to be the common denominator for activating secretory mechanisms, the direct involvement of cyclic AMP is still problematical and may even vary from organ to organ. Therefore, much work is still required to elucidate the exact nature of the role of cyclic AMP in the secretory mechanism.

But, on the basis of existing evidence, Rasmussen (Rasmussen and Nagata, 1970) developed a model to explain the interrelation between calcium and cyclic AMP. By considering various alternatives within the context of the messenger concept, he suggests the rather dubious possibility that cyclic AMP is the sole second messenger and that calcium may function in this system by simply being required for hormone–receptor interaction. An alternate proposal by Rasmussen involves the interaction of multiple second messengers, including both calcium and cyclic AMP. In this latter model, the two or more second messengers would be activated by stimulus–receptor interaction and act sequentially or in a parallel manner in the cell. This hypothetical sequence of cellular events accounts for some of the existing evidence, but it does not distinguish between whether the changes in calcium distribution and in adenylate cyclase activity are a simultaneous consequence of stimulus–receptor interaction or whether changes in adenylate cyclase lead to an increase in cyclic AMP which in turn brings about the translocation of calcium.

Although the purpose of this monograph has not been to provide a platform on which to espouse parochial views based solely on my own research, in conclusion I should like to present a model which has been developed in collaboration with two of my colleagues, Siret Jaanus and Richard Carchman, to explain the mechanism of ACTH action on the adrenal cortex. This model attempts to provide a unitary concept to account for the effects of calcium and cyclic AMP on the release response (Fig. 21).

Thus our investigations have established that, though an increase in adrenal activity cyclic AMP levels is associated with

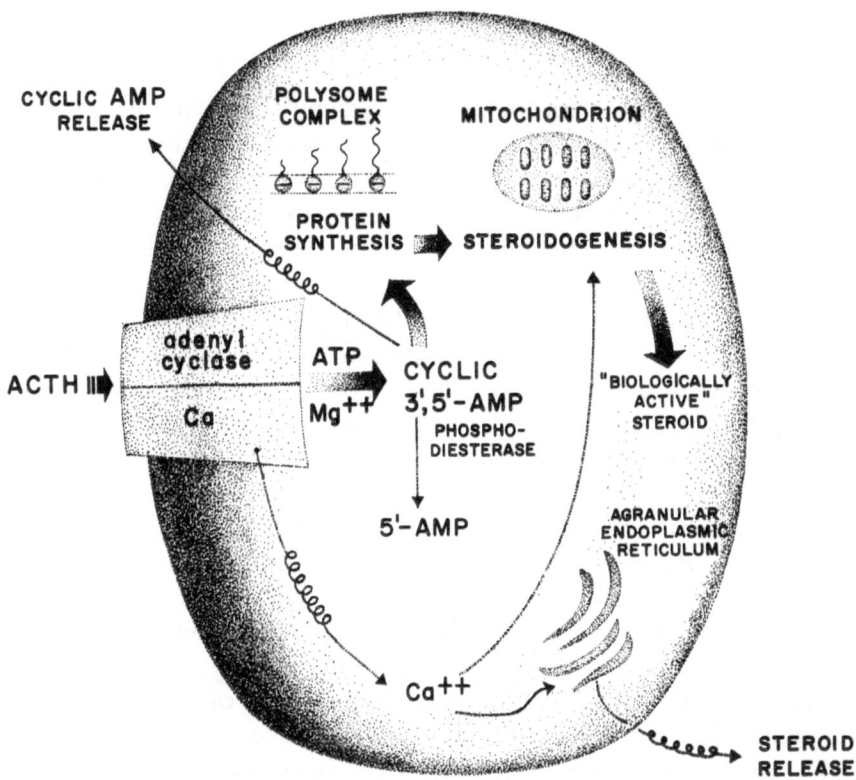

Fig. 21. Proposed model for action of ACTH on adrenal cortex. Interaction of ACTH with its receptor leads to a dissociation of calcium from its cyclase binding site. The resulting calcium mobilization causes an increase in adenylate cyclase activity, with a consequent rise in tissue cyclic AMP. The increase in cyclic nucleotide effects the formation or activation of some protein component, possibly a protein kinase, which leads to an increase in steroidogenesis within the mitochondria. The concomitant redistribution of calcium from its cyclase binding site to some locus within the interior of the cell (mitochondria or endoplasmic reticulum) triggers the release of the newly synthesized steroid (Rubin et al., 1972).

enhanced steroid synthesis and turnover in the perfused cat adrenal gland provided that calcium is present, an increase in cyclic AMP levels is not sufficient to trigger the physiological release response. These findings imply that the triggering of steroid release by ACTH involves an effect additional to simply activating adenylate cyclase and increasing cyclic AMP levels. The additional effect of ACTH appears to be a redistribution of cellular calcium which exogenous cyclic nucleotide cannot elicit (Rubin *et al.*, 1972).

Since perfusion with calcium-free solution greatly augments cyclase activity, and the effects of ACTH and calcium deprivation on augmenting cyclase activity and cyclic AMP levels are not additive, ACTH and calcium deprivation are probably activating cyclase by a similar mechanism. Thus these data are consistent with the model which proposes that, in the resting cortical cell, cyclase activity is kept at low levels by the presence of calcium and that ACTH activates cyclase by displacing this calcium fraction; the translocation of this fraction to the cell exterior may be responsible for initiating steroid release. This model thus affirms that changes in calcium distribution and in adenylate cyclase activity are simultaneous events and that cyclic AMP is not directly responsible for alterations in distribution of cellular calcium.

It should be emphasized that this hypothetical sequence of events has been elaborated solely on the basis of data obtained from the adrenal cortex; whether it has any applicability to other secretory systems remains to be determined. Needless to say, it is hoped that the more resourceful and imaginative researchers among us will eventually provide answers to such questions and to the other questions still to be answered. The most important of these involves not only the true interrelation between calcium and cyclic AMP but also whether their actions are fundamental to secretion by exocytosis. If this book provides the impetus for other investigators to confront these problems, then whatever efforts were expended in its preparation will have been worthwhile.

References

Abood, L. G. (1966), Interrelationships between phosphates and calcium in bioelectric phenomena, *Internat. Rev. Neurobiol. 9*: 223.

Abramson, M. B., Katzman, R., Wilson, C. E., and Gregor, H. P. (1964), Ionic properties of aqueous dispersions of phosphatidic acid, *J. Biol. Chem. 239*: 4066.

Ahn, C. S., and Rosenberg, I. N. (1970), Iodine metabolism in thyroid slices: Effects of TSH, dibutyryl cyclic 3'5'-AMP, NaF, and prostaglandin E_1, *Endocrinology 86*:396.

Allison, A. C. (1973), The role of microfilaments and microtubules in cell movement, endocytosis and exocytosis, in: *Locomotion of Tissue Cells*, Ciba Foundation Symposium, 14 (New Series), Elsevier, Amsterdam, p. 109.

Argent, B. E., Case, R. M., and Scratcherd, T. (1971), Stimulation of amylase secretion from the perfused cat pancreas by potassium and other alkali metal ions, *J Physiol. (London) 216*: 611.

Armstrong, P. B. (1966), On the role of metal cations in cellular adhesion: Effect on cell surface charge, *J. Exptl. Zool. 163*: 99.

Ashcroft, S. J. H., Hedeskov, C. J., and Randle, P. J. (1970), Glucose metabolism in mouse pancreatic islets, *Biochem. J. 118*: 143.

Ashley, C. C., and Ridgway, E. B. (1970), Aequorin–calcium luminescence and its application to muscle physiology, in: *Calcium and Cellular Function* (A. W. Cuthbert, ed.), Macmillan, London, p. 42.

Avioli, L. V., Shieber, W., and Kipnis, D. M. (1971), Role of glucagon and adrenergic receptors in thyrocalcitonin release in the dog, *Endocrinology 88*: 1337.

Babad, H., Ben-Zvi, R., Bdolah, A., and Schramm, H. (1967), The mechanism of enzyme secretion by the cell: 4. Effects of inducers, substrates and inhibitors on amylase secretion by rat parotid slices, *Europ. J. Biochem. 1*: 96.

151

Baker, P. F. (1972), Transport an metabolism of calcium ions in nerve, *Prog. Biophys. Mol. Biol. 24*: 177.

Banks, P. (1965), The adenosine-triphosphatase activity of adrenal chromaffin granules, *Biochem. J. 95*: 490.

Banks, P. (1966), An interaction between chromaffin granules and calcium ions, *Biochem. J. 101*: 18c.

Banks, P. (1967), The effect of ouabain on the secretion of catecholamines and on the intracellular concentration of potassium, *J. Physiol. (London) 193*: 631.

Banks, P. (1970), Involvement of calcium in the secretion of catecholamines, in: *Calcium and Cellular Function* (A. W. Cuthbert, ed.), Macmillan, London, p. 148.

Banks, P., and Helle, K. (1965), The release of protein from the stimulated adrenal medulla, *Biochem. J. 97*: 40c.

Banks, P., Mayor, D., Mitchell, M., and Tomlinson, D. (1971), Studies on the translocation of noradrenaline-containing vesicles in postganglionic sympathetic neurones *in vitro*: Inhibition of movement by colchicine and vinblastine and evidence for the involvement of axonal microtubules, *J. Physiol. (London) 216*: 625.

Barreras, R. F., and Donaldson, R. M. (1967), Effects of induced hypercalcemia on human gastric secretion, *Gastroenterology 52*: 670.

Basabe, J. C., Lopez, N. L., Viktora, J. K., and Wolff, F. W. (1971), Insulin secretion studied in the perfused rat pancreas. II. Effect of glucose, glucagon, 3',5'-adenosine monophosphate, theophylline, imidazole and phenoxybenzamine; their interaction with diazoxide, *Diabetes 20*: 457.

Bass, L., and Moore, W. J. (1966), Electrokinetic mechanism of miniature postsynaptic potentials, *Proc. Natl. Acad. Sci. 55*: 1214.

Batzri, S., and Selinger, Z. (1973), Enzyme secretion mediated by the epinephrine β-receptor in rat parotid slices, *J. Biol. Chem. 248*: 356.

Batzri, S., Amsterdam, A., Selinger, Z., Ohad, I., and Schramm, M. (1971), Epinephrine-induced vacuole formation in parotid gland cells and its independence of the secretory process, *Proc. Natl. Acad. Sci. 68*: 121.

Bauduin, H., Rochus, L., Vincent, D., and Dumont, J. E. (1971), Role of cyclic 3',5'-AMP in the action of physiological secretagogues on the metabolism of rat pancreas *in vitro*, *Biochim. Biophys. Acta 252*: 171.

Beall, R. J., and Sayers, G. (1972), Isolated adrenal cells: Steroidogenesis and cyclic AMP accumulation in response to ACTH, *Arch. Biochem. Biophys. 148*: 70.

Bell, N. H. (1970), Effects of glucagon, dibutyryl cyclic 3',5'-adenosine monophosphate and theophylline on calcitonin secretion *in vitro*, *J. Clin. Invest. 49*: 1368.

Bennett, L. L., Curry, D. L., and Grodsky, G. M. (1969), Calcium–magnesium antagonism in insulin secretion by the perfused rat pancreas, *Endocrinology 85*: 594.

Benz, L., Eckstein, B., Matthews, E. K., and Williams, J. A. (1972), Control of pancreatic amylase release *in vitro*: Effects of ions, cyclic AMP and colchicine, *Brit. J. Pharmacol. 46*: 66.

Bergström, S., Carlson, L. A., and Weeks, J. R. (1968), The prostaglandins: A family of biologically active lipids, *Pharmacol. Rev. 20*: 1.

Berl, S., Puszkin, S., and Nicklas, W. J. (1973), Actomyosin-like protein in brain, *Science 179*: 441.

Berlind, A., and Cooke, I. M. (1971), The role of divalent cations in electrically elicited release of a neurohormone from crab pericardial organs, *Gen. Comp. Endocrinol. 17*: 60.

Berneis, K. H., da Prada, M., and Pletscher, A. (1971), A possible mechanism for uptake of biogenic amines by storage organelles: Incorporation into nucleotide–metal aggregates, *Experientia 27*: 917.

Berridge, M. J., and Prince, W. T. (1972), The role of cyclic AMP in the control of fluid secretion, in: *Advances in Cyclic Nucleotide Research*, Vol. I, Raven Press, New York, p. 137.

Bettex-Galland, M., and Lüscher, E. F. (1965), Thrombostenin, the contractile protein from blood platelets and its relation to other contractile proteins, *Advan. Protein Chem. 20*: 1.

Bianchi, C. P. (1968), *Cell Calcium*, Appleton-Century-Crofts, New York.

Bieck, P. R. (1972), Role of cyclic AMP in the regulation of gastric secretion in dogs and humans, in: *Advances in Cyclic Nucleotide Research*, Vol. I, Raven Press, New York, p. 149.

Birks, R. I., and Cohen, M. W. (1968), The influence of internal sodium on the behavior of motor nerve endings, *Proc. Roy. Soc. (Ser. B, Biol. Sci.) 170*: 401.

Birmingham, M. K., Kurlents, E., Lane, R., Muhlstock, B., and Traikov, H. (1960), Effects of calcium on the potassium and sodium content of rat adrenal glands, on the stimulation of steroid production by adenosine 3',5'-monophosphate and on the response of the adrenal to short contact with ACTH, *Can. J. Biochem. Physiol. 38*: 1077.

Blaschko, H., and Welch, A. M. (1953), Localization of adrenaline in cytoplasmic particles of the bovine adrenal medulla, *Arch. Exptl. Pathol. Pharmakol. 219*: 17.

Blaschko, H., Comline, R. S., Schneider, F. H., Silver, M., and Smith, A. D. (1967), Secretion of a chromaffin granule protein, chromogranin, from the adrenal gland after splanchnic stimulation, *Nature 215*: 58.

Blaszkowski, T. P., and Bogdanski, D. F. (1971), Possible role of sodium and calcium ions in retention and physiological release of norepinephrine by adrenergic nerve endings, *Biochem. Pharmcol. 20*: 3281.

Blaustein, M. P. (1971), Preganglionic stimulation increases calcium uptake by sympathetic ganglia, *Science 172*: 391.

Blaustein, M. P., and Goldman, D. E. (1966), Competitive action of calcium and procaine on lobster axon, *J. Gen. Physiol. 49*: 1043.

Blaustein, M. P., and Goldman, D. E. (1968), The action of certain polyvalent cations on the voltage-clamped lobster axon, *J. Gen. Physiol. 51*: 279.

Blaustein, M. P., and Hodgkin, A. L. (1969), The effect of cyanide on the efflux of calcium from squid axons, *J. Physiol. (London) 200*: 497.

Blioch, Z. L., Glagoleva, I. M., Liberman, E. A., and Nenashev, V. A. (1968), A study of the mechanism of quantal transmitter release at a chemical synapse, *J. Physiol. (London) 199*: 11.

Boadle-Biber, M. C., Hughes, J., and Roth, R. H. (1970), Acceleration of noradrenaline biosynthesis in the guinea pig vas deferens by potassium, *Brit. J. Pharmacol. 40*: 702.

Bondani, A., and Karler, R. (1970), Interaction of calcium and local anesthetics with skeletal muscle microsomes, *J. Cell. Physiol. 75*: 199.

Borgeat, P., Chavancy, G., Dupont, A., Labrie, F., Arimura, A., and Schally, A. V. (1972), Stimulation of adenosine 3',5'-cyclic monophosphate accumulation in anterior pituitary gland *in vitro* by synthetic luteinizing hormone releasing hormone, *Proc. Natl. Acad. Sci. 69*: 2677.

Borle, A. (1967), Membrane transfer of calcium, *Clin. Orthop. Rel. Res. 52*: 267.

Borle, A. B. (1971), Calcium transport in kidney cells and its regulation, in: *Cellular Mechanisms for Calcium Transfer and Homeostasis* (G. Nichols and R. H. Wasserman, eds.), Academic Press, New York, p. 151.

Borowitz, J. L. (1970), Catecholamine binding complex in bovine adrenal medulla: Possible involvement of calcium, *Biochem. Pharmacol. 19*: 2475.

Borowitz, J. L. (1972), Effect of lanthanum on catecholamine release from adrenal medulla, *Life Sci. 11*: 959.

Borowitz, J. L., Fuwa, K., and Weiner, N. (1965), Distribution of metals and catecholamines in bovine adrenal medulla sub-cellular fractions, *Nature 205*: 42.

Boullin, D. J. (1967), The action of extracellular cations on the release of the sympathetic transmitter from peripheral nerves, *J. Physiol. (London) 189*: 85.

Bowers, C. Y. (1971), Studies on the role of cyclic AMP in the release of anterior pituitary hormones, *Ann. N.Y. Acad. Sci. 185*: 263.

Bracho, H., and Orkand, R. K. (1970), Effect of calcium on excitatory neuromuscular transmission in the crayfish, *J. Physiol. (London) 206*: 61.

Bressler, R., and Brendel, K. (1971), Effect of local anesthetics on insulin secretion by pancreas pieces, *Diabetes 20*: 721.

Bressler, R., Vargas-Cordon, M., and Lebovitz, H. E. (1968), Tranylcypromine: A potent insulin secretagogue and hypoglycemic agent, *Diabetes 17*: 617.

Brink, F. (1954), The role of calcium ions in neural processes, *Pharmacol. Rev. 6*: 243.

Brisson, G. R., Malaisse-Lagae, F., and Malaisse, W. J. (1972), The stimulus–secretion coupling of glucose-induced insulin release. VII. A proposed site of action for adenosine-3',5'-cyclic monophosphate, *J. Clin. Invest. 51*: 232.

Bulbring, E., and Tomita, T. (1970), Calcium and the action potential in smooth muscle, in: *Calcium and Cellular Function* (A. W. Cuthbert, ed.), Macmillan, London, p. 249.

Bull, R. J., and Trevor, A. J. (1972), Sodium and the flux of calcium ions in electrically-stimulated cerebral tissue, *J. Neurochem. 19*: 1011.

Brown, G. L., and Feldberg, W. (1936), The action of potassium on the superior cervical ganglion of the cat, *J. Physiol. (London) 86*: 290.

Burgen, A. S. V. (1956), The secretion of potassium in saliva, *J. Physiol. (London) 132*: 20.

Burke, G., Kowalski, K., and Yu, S. (1971), Effects of 3′,5′-cyclic nucleotides on membrane transport in isolated thyroid cells, *Acta Endocrinol. 68*: 183.

Burnside, B., and Manacek, F. J. (1972), Cytochalasin B: Problems in interpreting its effect on cells, *Develop. Biol. 27*: 443.

Bustos, G., and Roth, R. H. (1972), Release of monoamines from the striatum and hypothalamus: Effect of γ-hydroxybutyrate, *Brit. J. Pharmacol. 46*: 101.

Butcher, F. R., and Goldman, R. H. (1972), Effect of cytochalasin B and colchicine on the stimulation of γ-amylase release from rat parotid tissue slices, *Biochem. Biophys. Res. Commun. 48*: 23.

Carafoli, E., and Lehninger, A. L. (1971), A survey of the interaction of calcium ions with mitochondria from different tissues and species, *Biochem. J. 122*: 681.

Carafoli, E., Rossi, C. S., and Gazzotti, P. (1969), The effect of uncoupling agents and detergents on the movements of monovalent cations between mitochondria and medium, *Arch. Biochem. Biophys. 131*: 527.

Carchman, R. A., Jaanus, S. D., and Rubin, R. P. (1971), The role of adrenocorticotropin and calcium in adenosine cyclic 3′,5′-phosphate production and steroid release from the isolated perfused cat adrenal gland, *Mol. Pharmacol. 7*: 491.

Care, A. D., Cooper, C. W., Duncan, T., and Orimo, H. (1968), A study of thyrocalcitonin secretion by direct measurement of *in vivo* secretion rates in pigs, *Endocrinology 83*: 161.

Care, A. D., Bates, R. F. L., and Gitelman, H. J. (1971a), Evidence for a role of cyclic AMP in the release of calcitonin, *Ann. N.Y. Acad. Sci. 185*: 317.

Care, A. D., Bell, N. H., and Bates, R. F. L. (1971b), The effects of hypermagnesemia on calcitonin secretion *in vivo*, *J. Endocrinol. 51*: 381.

Carlsson, A., Hillarp, N. A., and Hökfelt, B. (1957), The concomitant release of adenosine triphosphate and catechol amines from the adrenal medulla, *J. Biol. Chem. 227*: 243.

Carr, C. W., and Chang, K. Y. (1971), The binding of calcium with nucleic acids and phospholipids, in: *Cellular Mechanisms for Calcium Transfer and Homeostasis* (G. Nichols and R. N. Wasserman, eds.), Academic Press, New York, p. 41.

Carvalho, A. P. (1966), Binding of cations by microsomes from rabbit skeletal muscle, *J. Cell. Physiol. 67*: 73.

Case, R. M., and Clausen, T. (1971), Stimulus–secretion coupling in exocrine pancreas. II. The role of calcium ions, in: *Proceedings of the Vth Scandinavian Conference on Gastroenterology*, Centraltrykkeriet, Ålborg, p. 67.

Case, R. M., and Scratcherd, T. (1972a), The actions of dibutyryl cyclic adenosine 3′,5′-monophosphate and methyl xanthines on pancreatic exocrine secretion, *J. Physiol. (London) 223*: 649.

Case, R. M., and Scratcherd, T. (1972b), Prostaglandin action on pancreatic blood flow and on electrolyte and enzyme secretion by exocrine pancreas *in vivo* and *in vitro, J. Physiol. (London) 226*: 393.

Case, R. M., Johnson, M., Scratcherd, T., and Sherratt, H. S. A. (1972), Cyclic adenosine 3′,5′-monophosphate concentration in the pacreas following stimulation by secretin, cholecystokinin-pancreozymin and acetylcholine, *J. Physiol. (London) 223*: 669.

Chakravarty, N. (1962), Inhibition of anaphylactic histamine release by 2-deoxyglucose, *Nature 194*: 1182.

Chance, B. (1965), The energy-linked reaction of calcium with mitochondria, *J. Biol. Chem. 240*: 2729.

Chapman, R. A., and Niedergerke, R. (1970), Interaction between heart rate and calcium concentration in the control of contractile strength of the frog heart, *J. Physiol. (London) 211*: 423.

Charles, M. A., Fanska, R., Schmid, F. G., Forsham, P. H., and Grodsky, G. M. (1973), Adenosine 3′,5′-monophosphate in pancreatic islets: Glucose-induced insulin release, *Science 179*: 569.

Cheng, K. W., Martin, J. B., and Friesen, H. (1972), Studies of neurophysin release, *Endocrinology 91*: 177.

Chubb, I. W., DePotter, W. P., and DeSchaepdryver, A. F. (1972), Tyramine does not release noradrenaline from splenic nerve by exocytosis, *Naunyn-Schmiedebergs Arch. Pharmakol. 274*: 281.

Collier, B. (1969), The preferential release of newly synthesized transmitter by a sympathetic ganglion, *J. Physiol. (London) 205*: 341.

Colomo, F., and Erulkar, S. D. (1968), Miniature synaptic potentials at frog spinal neurones in the presence of tetrodotoxin, *J. Physiol. (London) 199*: 205.

Colomo, F., and Rahamimoff, R. (1968), Interaction between sodium and calcium ions in the process of transmitter release at the neuromuscular junction, *J. Physiol. (London) 198*: 203.

Cooke, J. D., Okamoto, K., and Quastel, D. M. J. (1973), The role of calcium in depolarization–secretion coupling at the motor nerve terminal, *J. Physiol. (London) 228*: 459.

Cooke, S. A. R. (1971), The distribution of calcium in the human kidney: Method and results, *Brit. J. Urol. 43*: 130.

Cooke, W. J., and Robinson, J. D. (1971), Factors influencing calcium movements in rat brain slices, *Am. J. Physiol. 221*: 218.

Coombs, J. S., Eccles, J. C., and Fatt, P. (1955), The specific ionic conductances and the ionic movement across the motoneuronal membrane that produce the inhibitory postsynaptic potential, *J. Physiol. (London) 130*: 326.

Copp, D. H. (1969), Calcitonin and parathyroid hormone, *Ann. Rev. Pharmacol.* 9: 327.

Copp, D. H. (1970), Endocrine regulation of calcium metabolism, *Ann. Rev. Physiol. 32*: 61.

Cosmos, E., and Harris, E. J. (1961), *In vitro* studies of the gain and exchange of calcium in frog skeletal muscle, *J. Gen. Physiol. 44*: 1121.

Coupland, R. E. (1965), *The Natural History of the Chromaffin Cell*, Longmans, Green, London.

Cramer, W. (1928), *Fever, Heat Regulation, Climate and the Thyroid–Adrenal Apparatus*, Longmans, Green, London.

Curran, P. F., and Gill, J. R. (1962), The effect of calcium on sodium transport by frog skin, *J. Gen. Physiol. 45*: 625.

Curry, D. L., Bennett, L. L., and Grodsky, G. M. (1968a), Requirement for calcium ion in insulin secretion by the perfused rat pancreas, *Am. J. Physiol. 214*: 174.

Curry, D. L., Bennett, L. L., and Grodsky, G. M. (1968b), Dynamics of insulin secretion by the perfused rat pancreas, *Endocrinology 83*: 572.

Cuthbert, A. W. (1967), Membrane lipids and drug action, *Pharmacol. Rev. 19*: 59.

Dahlquist, R., and Diamant, B. (1972), Relation of uptake of sodium and calcium to ATP-induced histamine release from rat mast cells, in: *Fifth International Congress on Pharmacology* (San Francisco, July 23–28), p. 50 (abst.).

Dahlstrom, A. (1970), The effects of drugs on axonal transport of amine storage granules, in: *New Aspects of Storage and Release Mechanisms of Catecholamines*, Bayer Symposium II (H. J. Schümann and G. Kroneberg, eds.), Springer, New York, p. 20.

Davey, M. G., and Lüscher, E. F. (1968), Release reactions of human platelets induced by thrombin and other agents, *Biochim. Biophys. Acta 165*: 490.

Davson, H., and Danielli, J. F. (1952), *The Permeability of Natural Membranes*, 2nd ed., Cambridge University Press, London.

Dawson, R. M. C., and Hauser, H. (1970), Binding of calcium to phospholipids, in: *Calcium and Cellular Function* (A. W. Cuthbert, ed.), Macmillan, London, p. 17.

Dean, C. R., and Hope, D. B. (1968), The isolation of neurophysin I and II from bovine pituitary neurosecretory granules separated on a large scale from other subcellular organelles, *Biochem. J. 106*: 565.

Dean, P. M., and Matthews, E. K. (1968), Electrical activity in pancreatic islet cells, *Nature 219*: 389.

Dean, P. M., and Matthews, E. K. (1970a), Glucose-induced electrical activity in pancreatic islet cells, *J. Physiol. (London) 210*: 255.

Dean, P. M., and Matthews, E. K. (1970b), Electrical activity in pancreatic islet cells: Effects of ions, *J. Physiol. (London) 210*: 265.

DeBassio, W. A., Schnitzler, R. M., and Parsons, R. L. (1971), Influence of lanthanum on transmitter release at the neuromuscular junction, *J. Neurobiol. 2*: 263.

Dekker, A., and Field, J. B. (1970), Correlation of effects of thyrotropin, prostaglandins and ions on glucose oxidation, cyclic AMP, and colloid droplet formation in dog thyroid slices, *Metabolism 19*: 453.

Del Castillo, J., and Katz, B. (1954), The effect of magnesium on the activity of motor nerve endings, *J. Physiol. (London) 124*: 553.

Del Castillo, J., and Katz, B. (1956), Biophysical aspects of neuromuscular transmission, *Prog. Biophys. Mol. Biol. 6*: 121.

DeRobertis, E. (1959), Submicroscopic morphology of the synapse, *Internat. Rev. Cytol. 8*: 61.

DeRobertis, E. D. P., and Bennett, H. S. (1955), Some features of the submicroscopic morphology of synapses in frog and earthworm, *J. Biophys. Biochem. Cytol. 1*: 47.

DeRobertis, E. D. P., and VazFerreira, A. (1957), Electron microscope study of the excretion of catechol-containing droplets in the adrenal medulla, *Exptl. Cell Res. 12*: 568.

Diamant, B., and Krüger, P. G. (1967), Histamine release from isolated rat peritoneal mast cells induced by adenosine-5′ triphosphate, *Acta Physiol. Scand. 71*: 291.

Diamant, B., and Peterson, C. (1970), The effect of glucose on histamine release from isolated rat peritoneal mast cells induced by adenosine-5′-triphosphate, *Acta Physiol. Scand. 80*: 299.

Diamant, B., and Uvnäs, B. (1961), Evidence for energy-requiring processes in histamine release and mast cell degranulation in rat tissue induced by compound 48/80, *Acta Physiol. Scand. 53*: 315.

Diamond, I., and Goldberg, A. L. (1971), Uptake and release of ^{45}Ca by brain microsomes, synaptosomes, and synaptic vesicles, *J. Neurochem. 18*: 1419.

Dicker, S. E. (1966), Release of vasopressin and oxytocin from isolated pituitary glands of adult and new-born rats, *J. Physiol. (London) 185*: 429.

Dodge, F. A., and Rahamimoff, R. (1967), Cooperative action of calcium ions in transmitter release at the neuromuscular junction, *J. Physiol. (London) 193*: 419.

Dodge, F. A., Miledi, R., and Rahamimoff, R. (1969), Strontium and quantal release of transmitter at the neuromuscular junction, *J. Physiol. (London) 200*: 267.

Douglas, W. W. (1965), Acetylcholine as a secretogogue: Calcium-dependent links in stimulus–secretion coupling at the adrenal medulla and submaxillary gland, in: *Pharmacology of Cholinergic and Adrenergic Transmission* (G. B. Koelle, W. W. Douglas, and A. Carlsson, eds.), Pergamon Press, New York, p. 95.

Douglas, W. W. (1968), Stimulus–secretion coupling: The concept and clues from chromaffin and other cells, *Brit. J. Pharmacol. 34*: 451.

Douglas, W. W., and Ishida, A. (1965), The stimulant effect of cold on vasopressin release from the neurohypophysis *in vitro*, *J. Physiol. (London) 179*: 185.

Douglas, W. W., and Kanno, T. (1967), The effect of amethocaine on acetyl-choline-induced depolarization and catecholamine secretion in the adrenal chromaffin cell, *Brit. J. Pharmacol. 30*: 612.

Douglas, W. W., and Poisner, A. M. (1962), On the mode of acetylcholine in evoking adrenal medullary secretion: Increased uptake of calcium during the secretory response, *J. Physiol. (London) 162*: 385.

Douglas, W. W., and Poisner, A. M. (1963), The influence of calcium on the secretory response of the submaxillary gland to acetylcholine or to norad-renaline, *J. Physiol. (London) 165*: 528.

Douglas, W. W., and Poisner, A. M. (1964a), Stimulus–secretion coupling in a neurosecretory organ: The role of calcium in the release of vasopressin from the neurohypophysis, *J. Physiol. (London) 172*: 1.

Douglas, W. W., and Poisner, A. M. (1964b), Calcium movement in the neurohypophysis of the rat and its relation to the release of vasopressin, *J. Physiol. (London) 172*: 19.

Douglas, W. W., and Rubin, R. P. (1961), The role of calcium in the secretory response of the adrenal medulla to acetylcholine, *J. Physiol. (London) 159*: 40.

Douglas, W. W., and Rubin, R. P. (1963), The mechanism of catecholamine release from the adrenal medulla and the role of calcium in stimulus–secretion coupling, *J. Physiol. (London) 167*: 288.

Douglas, W. W., and Rubin, R. P. (1964a), The effects of alkaline earths and other divalent cations on adrenal medullary secretion, *J. Physiol. (London) 175*: 231.

Douglas, W. W., and Rubin, R. P. (1964b), Stimulant action of barium on the adrenal medulla, *Nature 203*: 305.

Douglas, W. W., and Sorimachi, M. (1971), Electrically evoked release of vasopressin from isolated neurohypophyses in sodium-free media, *Brit. J. Pharmacol. 42*: 647P.

Douglas, W. W., and Sorimachi, M. (1972a), Effects of cytochalasin B and colchicine on secretion of posterior pituitary and adrenal medullary hor-mones. *Brit. J. Pharmacol. 45*: 143P.

Douglas, W. W., and Sorimachi, M. (1972b), Colchicine inhibits adrenal medul-lary secretion evoked by acetylcholine without affecting that evoked by potassium, *Brit. J. Pharmacol. 45*: 129.

Douglas, W. W., Lywood, D. W., and Straub, R. W. (1961), The stimulant effect of barium on the release of acetylcholine from the superior cervical ganglion, *J. Physiol. (London) 156*: 515.

Douglas, W. W., Ishida, A., and Poisner, A. M. (1965), The effects of metabolic inhibitors on the release of vasopressin from the isolated neurohypophysis, *J. Physiol. (London) 181*: 753.

Douglas, W. W., Kanno, T., and Sampson, S. (1967a), Effects of acetylcholine and other medullary secretogogues and antagonists on the membrane potential of adrenal chromaffin cells: An analysis employing techniques of tissue culture, *J. Physiol. (London) 188*: 107.

Douglas, W. W., Kanno, T., and Sampson, S. (1967b), Influence of the ionic environment on the membrane potential of the adrenal chromaffin cells and on the depolarizing effect of acetylcholine, *J. Physiol. (London) 191*: 107.

Douglas, W. W., Nagasawa, J., and Schulz, R. (1970), Electron microscopic studies on the mechanism of secretion of posterior pituitary hormones and significance of microvesicles ("synaptic vesicles"): Evidence of secretion by exocytosis and formation of microvesicles as a byproduct of this process, in: *Memoirs of the Society for Endocrinology*, No. 19: *Subcellular Organization and Function in Endocrine Tissues* (H. Heller and K. Lederis, eds.), Cambridge University Press, London, p. 353.

Dransfeld, H., Greeff, K., Schorn, A., and Ting, B. T. (1969), Calcium uptake in mitochondria and vesicles of heart and skeletal muscle in presence of potassium, sodium, K-strophanthin and pentobarbital, *Biochem. Pharmacol. 18*: 1335.

Dreifuss, J. J., Kalnins, I., Kelly, J. S., and Ruf, K. B. (1971), Action potentials and release of neurohypophysial hormones *in vitro*, *J. Physiol. (London) 215*: 805.

Dreisbach, R. H. (1964), Calcium transfer in salivary and lacrimal glands, in: *Salivary Glands and Their Secretions* (L. M. Sreebny and J. Meyer, eds.), Pergamon Press, Oxford, p. 237.

Droller, M. J., and Wolfe, S. M. (1972), Thrombin-induced increase in intracellular cyclic $3',5'$-adenosine monophosphate in human platelets, *J. Clin. Invest. 51*: 3094.

Dumont, J. E., Willems, C., Van Sande, J., and Nève, P. (1971), Regulation of the release of thyroid hormones: Role of cyclic AMP, *Ann. N. Y. Acad. Sci. 185*: 291.

Dumont, P. A., Curran, P. F., and Solomon, A. K. (1960), Calcium and strontium in rat small intestine: Their fluxes and their effect on Na flux, *J. Gen. Physiol. 43*: 1119.

Dunham, E. T., and Glynn, I. M. (1961), Adenosine triphosphatase activity and the active movements of alkali metal ions, *J. Physiol. (London) 156*: 274.

Ebashi, S. (1972), Calcium ions and muscle contraction, *Nature 240*: 217.

Ebashi, S., and Endo, M. (1968), Calcium ion and muscle contraction, *Prog. Biophys. 18*: 125.

Edman, K. A. P., and Schild, H. O. (1962), The need for calcium in the responses induced by acetylcholine and potassium in the rat uterus, *J. Physiol. (London) 161*: 424.

Engbaek, L. (1952), The pharmacological actions of magnesium ions with particular reference to the neuromuscular and cardiovascular system, *Pharmacol. Rev. 4*: 396.

Entman, M. L., Levey, G. S., and Epstein, S. E. (1969), Mechanism of action of epinephrine and glucagon on the canine heart: Evidence for increase in sarcotubular calcium stores mediated by cyclic $3',5'$-AMP, *Circ. Res. 25*: 429.

Estensen, R. D., and Plagemann, P. G. W. (1972), Cytochalasin B: Inhibition of glucose and glucosamine transport, *Proc. Natl. Acad. Sci. 69*: 1430.

Farese, R. V. (1971), On the requirement for calcium during the steroidogenic effect of ACTH, *Endocrinology 89*: 1057.

Fatt, P., and Ginsborg, B. L. (1958), The ionic requirements for the production of action potentials in crustacean muscle fibres, *J. Physiol. (London) 142*: 516.

Fawcett, C. P., Powell, A. E., and Sachs, H. (1968), Biosynthesis and release of neurophysin, *Endocrinology 83*: 1299.

Fawcett, D. W., Long, J. A., and Jones, A. L. (1969), The ultrastructure of endocrine glands, *Rec. Prog. Horm. Res. 25*: 315.

Feinblatt, J. D., and Raisz, L. G. (1971), Secretion of thyrocalcitonin in organ cultures, *Endocrinology 88*: 797.

Feinstein, M. B. (1964), Reaction of local anesthetics with phospholipids: A possible chemical basis for anesthesia, *J. Gen. Physiol. 48*: 357.

Feinstein, M. B. (1966), Inhibition of contraction and calcium exchangeability in the rat uterus by local anesthetics, *J. Pharmacol. Exptl. Therap. 52*: 516.

Field, J., Dekker, A., Zor, U., and Kaneko, T. (1971), Conference on Prostaglandins, *Proc. N.Y. Acad. Sci. 180*: 268.

Fillenz, M. (1971), Fine structure of noradrenaline storage vesicles in nerve terminals of the rat vas deferens, *Phil. Trans. Roy. Soc. London B 261*: 319.

Fillion, G., Nosal, R., and Uvnäs, B. (1971), The presence of a sulphomucopolysaccharide–protein complex in adrenal medullary cell granules, *Acta Physiol. Scand. 83*: 286.

Fillion, G. M. B., Slorach, S. A., and Uvnäs, B. (1970), The release of histamine, heparin, and granule protein from rat mast cells treated with compound 48/80 *in vitro*, *Acta Physiol. Scand. 78*: 547.

Flack, J. D. (1974), The hypothalamus–pituitary–endocrine system, in: *The Prostaglandins*, Vol. I (P. W. Ramwell, ed.), Plenum Press, New York, p. 327.

Flack, J. D., and Ramwell, P. W. (1972), A comparison of the effects of ACTH, cyclic AMP, dibutyryl cyclic AMP, and PGE_2 on corticosteroidogenesis *in vitro*, *Endocrinology 90*: 371.

Fleischer, N., Donald, R. A., and Butcher, R. W. (1969), Involvement of adenosine 3′,5′-monophosphate in release of ACTH, *Am. J. Physiol. 217*: 1287.

Ford, L. E., and Podolsky, R. J. (1972), Intracellular calcium movements in skinned muscle fibres, *J. Physiol. (London) 223*: 21.

Foreman, J. C., and Mongar, J. L. (1972), The role of the alkaline earth ions in anaphylactic histamine secretion, *J. Physiol. (London) 224*: 753.

Forstner, J., and Manery, J. F. (1971), Calcium binding by human erythrocyte membranes, *Biochem. J. 124*: 563.

Forte, J. G., and Nauss, A. H. (1963), Effects of calcium removal on bullfrog gastric mucosa, *Am. J. Physiol. 205*: 631.

Forte, J. G., Forte, T. M., and Ray, T. K. (1972), Membranes of the oxyntic cell: Their structure, composition and genesis, in: *Gastric Secretion* (G. Sachs, E. Heinz, and K. J. Ullrich, eds.), Academic Press, New York, p. 37.

Frank, G. B. (1962), Utilization of bound calcium in the action of caffeine and certain multivalent cations on skeletal muscle, *J. Physiol. (London) 163*: 254.

Frankenhaeuser, B., and Hodgkin, A. L. (1957), The action of calcium on the electrical properties of squid axons, *J. Physiol. (London) 137*: 218.

Frankenhaeuser, B., and Meves, H. (1958), The effect of magnesium and calcium on the frog myelinated nerve fiber, *J. Physiol. (London) 147*: 360.

Furchgott, R. F. (1960), Spiral cut strip of rabbit aorta for *in vitro* studies of arterial smooth muscle, *Meth. Med. Res. 8*: 177.

Gage, P. W. (1967), Depolarization and excitation–secretion coupling in presynaptic terminals, *Fed. Proc. 26*: 1627.

Gage, P. W., and Quastel, D. M. J. (1965), Dual effect of potassium in transmitter release, *Nature 206*: 625.

Garren, L. D., Gill, G. N., Masui, H., and Walton, G. M. (1971), On the mechanism of action of ACTH, *Rec. Prog. Horm. Res. 27*: 433.

Geffen, L. B., Livett, B. G., and Rush, R. A. (1970), Immunohistochemical localization of chromogranins in sheep sympathetic neurones and their release by nerve impulses, in: *New Aspects of Storage and Release Mechanisms of Catecholamines*, Bayer Symposium II (H. J. Schümann and G. Kroneberg, eds.), Springer, New York, p. 58.

Geschwind, I. I. (1969), Mechanism of action of releasing factors, in: *Frontiers in Neuroendocrinology* (W. F. Ganong and L. Martini, eds.), Oxford University Press, New York, p. 389.

Geschwind, I. I. (1970), Mechanism of action of hypothalamic adenohypophysiotropic factors, in: *Hypophysiotropic Hormones of the Hypothalamus.* (J. Meites, ed.), Williams and Wilkins, Baltimore, p. 298.

Gillespie, E. (1971), Colchicine binding in tissue slices: Decrease by calcium and biphasic effect of adenosine-3',5'-monophosphate, *J. Cell. Biol. 50*: 544.

Gillespie, E., Levine, R. J., and Malawista, S. (1968), Histamine release from rat peritoneal mast cells: Inhibition by colchicine and potentiation by deuterium oxide, *J. Pharmacol. Exptl. Therap. 164*: 158.

Gilman, A. G., and Rall, T. W. (1968), The role of adenosine-3',5'-phosphate in mediating effects of thyroid-stimulating hormone on carbohydrate metabolism of bovine thyroid slices, *J. Biol. Chem. 243*: 5872.

Gingell, D., Garrod, D. R., and Palmer, J. F. (1970), Divalent cations and cell adhesion, in: *Calcium and Cellular Function* (A. W. Cuthbert, ed.), Macmillan, London, p. 59.

Ginsborg, B. L., and Hirst, G. D. S. (1972), The effect of adenosine on the release of the transmitter from the phrenic nerve of the rat, *J. Physiol. (London) 224*: 629.

Ginsburg, M. (1968), Molecular aspects of neurohypophysial hormone release, *Proc. Roy. Soc. (Ser. B, Sci.) 170*: 27.

Goldberg, A. L., and Singer, J. J. (1969), Evidence for a role of cyclic AMP in neuromuscular transmission, *Proc. Natl. Acad. Sci. 64*: 134.

Goodford, P. J. (1967), The calcium content of the smooth muscle of the guinea pig taenia coli, *J. Physiol. (London), 192*: 145.

Goodman, D. B. P., Rasmussen, H., DiBella, F., and Guthrow, C. E. (1970), Cyclic adenosine 3',5'-monophosphate-stimulated phosphorylation of isolated neurotubule units, *Proc. Natl. Acad. Sci. 67*: 652.

Grahame-Smith, D. G., Butcher, R. W., Ney, R. L., and Sutherland, E. W. (1967), Adenosine 3',5'-monophosphate as the intracellular mediator of the action of adrenocorticotropic hormone on the adrenal cortex, *J. Biol. Chem. 242*: 5535.

Gray, J. S., and Adkinson, J. L. (1941), The effect of inorganic ions on gastric secretion *in vitro, Am. J. Physiol. 134*: 27.

Grette, K. (1962), Studies on the mechanism of thrombin-catalyzed hemostatic reactions in blood platelets, *Acta Physiol. Scand. 56* (Suppl. 195): 1.

Grodsky, G. M. (1970), Insulin and the pancreas, *Vit. Horm. 28*: 37.

Gross, P. R. (1954), On the mechanism of the yolk-lysis reaction, *Protoplasma 43*: 416.

Grossman, A., and Furchgott, R. F. (1964), The effects of external calcium concentration on the distribution and exchange of calcium in resting and beating guinea pig auricles, *J. Pharmacol. Exptl. Therap. 143*: 107.

Grynszpan-Winograd, O. (1971), Morphological aspects of exocytosis in the adrenal medulla, *Phil. Trans. Roy. Soc. London B 261*: 291.

Guidotti, A., and Costa, E. (1973), Involvement of adenosine 3',5'-monophosphate in the activation of tyrosine hydroxylase elicited by drugs, *Science 179*: 902.

Guttman, R. (1940), Stabilization of spider crab nerve membrane by alkaline earths as manifested in resting potential measurements, *J. Gen. Physiol. 23*: 343.

Hagiwara, S., and Nakajima, S. (1966), Differences in Na and Ca spikes as examined by application of tetrodotoxin, procaine and manganese ions, *J. Gen. Physiol. 49*: 793.

Hagiwara, S., and Takahashi, K. (1967), Surface density of calcium ions and calcium spikes in the barnacle muscle fiber membrane, *J. Gen. Physiol. 50*: 583.

Haksar, A., and Peron, F. G. (1972), Comparison of the Ca^{++} requirement for the steroidongenic effect of ACTH and dibutyryl cyclic AMP in rat adrenal cell suspensions, *Biochem. Biophys. Res. Commun. 47*: 445.

Hales, C. N. (1971), Ionic investigations of the mechanism of insulin secretion, in: *Subcellular Organization and Function in Endocrine Tissues* (H. Heller and K. Lederis, eds.), Memoirs of the Society for Endocrinology, Vol. 19, Cambridge University Press, London, p. 397.

Hales, C. N., and Miller, R. D. G. (1968a), The role of sodium and potassium in insulin secretion from rabbit pancreas, *J. Physiol. (London) 194*: 725.

Hales, C. N., and Milner, R. D. G. (1968b), Cations and the secretion of insulin from rabbit pancreas *in vitro, J. Physiol. (London) 199*: 177.

Hamilton, J. W., and Cohn, D. V. (1969), Studies on the biosynthesis *in vitro* of parathyroid hormone. I. Synthesis of parathyroid hormone by bovine parathyroid gland slices and its control by calcium, *J. Biol. Chem. 244*: 5421.

Harris, J. B., and Alonso, D. (1965), Stimulation of the gastric mucosa by adenosine 3',5'-monophosphate, *Fed. Proc. 24*: 1368.

Harrison, D. G., and Long, C. (1968), The calcium content of human erythrocytes, *J. Physiol. (London) 199*: 367.

Harvey, A. M., and MacIntosh,.F. C. (1940), Calcium and synaptic transmission in a sympathetic ganglion, *J. Physiol. (London) 97*: 408.

Hedge, G. (1971), ACTH secretion due to hypothalamo-pituitary effects of adenosine 3',5'-monophosphate and related substances, *Endocrinology 89*: 500.

Hedge, G. (1972), The effects of prostaglandins on ACTH secretion, *Endocrinology 91*: 925.

Hedqvist, P. (1970), Studies on the effect of prostaglandins E_1 and E_2 on the sympathetic neuromuscular transmission in some animal tissues, *Acta Physiol. Scand. Suppl. 345*: 1.

Heilbrunn, L. V. (1956), *The Dynamics of Living Protoplasm*, Academic Press, New York.

Heisler, S., Fast, D., and Tenenhouse, A. (1972), Role of Ca^{++} and cyclic AMP in protein secretion from rat exocrine pancreas, *Biochim. Biophys. Acta 279*: 561.

Helander, H. F. (1967), Light and electron microscopy of the gastric mucosa, in: *The Physiology of Gastric Secretion* (L. S. Semb and J. Myren, eds.), Williams and Wilkins, Baltimore, p. 58.

Helander, H. F., Sanders, S. S., Rehm, W. S., and Hirschowitz, B. I. (1972), Quantitative aspects of gastric morphology, in: *Gastric Secretion* (G. Sachs, E. Heinz, and K. J. Ullrich, eds.), Academic Press, New York, p. 69.

Hellman, B., Sehlin, J., and Täljedal, I. B. (1971), Calcium uptake by pancreatic μ cells as measured with the aid of ^{45}Ca and mannitol-^3H, *Am. J. Physiol. 221*: 1795.

Hertelendy, F. (1971), Studies on growth hormone secretion. II. Stimulation by prostaglandins *in vitro*, *Acta Endocrinol. 68*: 355.

Heuser, J., and Miledi, R. (1971), Effect of lanthanum ions on function and structure of frog neuromuscular junctions, *Proc. Roy. Soc. (Ser. B, Biol. Sci.) 179*: 247.

Hillarp, N. A. (1959), Further observations on the state of the catecholamines stored in the adrenal medullary granules, *Acta Physiol. Scand. 47*: 271.

Hillarp, N. A. (1960), Different pools of catecholamines stored in the adrenal medulla, *Acta Physiol. Scand. 50*: 8.

Hillarp, N. A., and Thieme, G. (1959), Nucleotides in the catecholamine granules of the adrenal medulla, *Acta Physiol. Scand. 45*: 328.

Hillarp, N. A., Langerstedt, S., and Nilson, B. (1953), The isolation of a granular fraction from the suprarenal medulla containing the sympathetic catecholamines, *Acta Physiol. Scand. 29*: 251.

Hille, B. (1970), Ionic channels in nerve membranes, *Prog. Biophys. Mol. Biol. 21*: 1.

Hilmy, M. I., and Somjen, G. G. (1968), Distribution and tissue uptake of magnesium related to its pharmacological effects, *Am. J. Physiol. 214*: 406.

Hirsch, P. F., and Munson, P. L. (1969), Thyrocalcitonin, *Physiol. Rev. 49*: 548.

Höber, R. (1945), *Physical Chemistry of Cells and Tissues*, Blakiston, Philadelphia.

Hodgkin, A. L., and Katz, B. (1949a), The effect of sodium ions on the electrical activity of the giant axon of the squid, *J. Physiol. (London), 108*: 37.

Hodgkin, A. L., and Katz, B. (1949b), The effect of calcium on the axoplasm of giant nerve fibers, *J. Exptl. Biol. 26*: 292.

Hodgkin, A. L., and Keynes, R. D. (1957), Movements of labelled calcium in squid giant axons, *J. Physiol. (London), 138*: 253.

Hofmann, W. W., Struppler, A., Weindl, A., and Velho, F. (1973), Neuromuscular transmission with colchicine-treated nerves, *Brain Res. 49*: 208.

Hokin, L. E. (1966), Effects of calcium omission on acetylcholine-stimulated amylase secretion and phospholipid synthesis in pigeon pancreas slice, *Biochim. Biophys. Acta 115*: 219.

Holmsen, H., and Day, H. J. (1970), The selectivity of the thrombin-induced platelet release reaction: Subcellular localization of released and retained constituents, *J. Lab. Clin. Med. 75*: 840.

Holmsen, H., Day, H. J., and Stormken, H. (1969), The blood platelet release reaction, *Scand. J. Hematol. Suppl. 8*: 1.

Holmsen, H., Day, H. J., and Setkowsky, C. (1972), Secretory mechanisms: Behaviour of adenine nucleotides during the platelet release reaction induced by adenosine diphosphate and adrenaline, *Biochem. J. 129*: 67.

Hoyle, G. (1955), The effects of some common cations on neuromuscular transmission in insects, *J. Physiol (London) 127*: 90.

Hubbard, J. I. (1970), Mechanism of transmitter release, *Prog, Biophys. Mol. Biol. 21*: 33.

Hubbard, J. I., and Kwanbunbumpen, S. (1968), Evidence for the vesicle hypothesis, *J. Physiol. (London) 194*: 407.

Huković, S., and Muscholl, E. (1962), Die Noradrenalin: Abgabe aus dem isolierten Kaninchenherzen bei sympathischen Nervenreizung und ihre pharmakologische Beeinflussung, *Naunyn-Schmiedebergs Arch. Pharmakol. 244*: 81.

Hutter, O. F., and Kostial, K. (1954), Effect of magnesium and calcium ions on the release of acetylcholine, *J. Physiol. (London) 124*: 234.

Hutter, O. F., and Kostial, K. (1955), The relationship of sodium ions to the release of acetylcholine, *J. Physiol. (London) 129*: 159.

Ishida, H., Miki, N., and Yoshida, H. (1971), Role of Ca^{++} in the secretion of amylase from the parotid gland, *Jap. J. Pharmacol. 21*: 227.

Jaanus, S. D., and Rubin, R. P. (1971), The effect of ACTH on calcium distribution in the perfused cat adrenal gland, *J. Physiol. 213*: 581.

Jaanus, S. D., Rosenstein, M. J., and Rubin, R. P. (1970), On the mode of action of ACTH on the isolated perfused adrenal gland, *J. Physiol. (London) 209*: 539.

Jacobson, A., Schwartz, M., and Rehm, W. S. (1965), Effects of removal of calcium from bathing media on frog stomach, *Am. J. Physiol. 209*: 134.

Jahn, T. L., and Bovee, E. C. (1969), Protoplasmic movements within cells, *Physiol. Rev. 49*: 793.

Jamieson, J. D., and Palade, G. E. (1967), Intracellular transport of secretory proteins in the pancreatic exocrine cell. II. Transport to condensing vacuoles and zymogen granules, *J. Cell Biol. 34*: 597.

Jenkinson, D. H. (1957), The nature of the antagonism between calcium and magnesium ions at the neuromuscular junction, *J. Physiol. (London) 138*: 434.

Johnson, D. G., Thoa, N. B., Weinshilboum, R., Axelrod, J., and Kopin, I. J. (1971), Enhanced release of dopamine-β-hydroxylase from sympathetic nerves by calcium and phenoxybenzamine and its reversal by prostaglandins, *Proc. Natl. Acad. Sci. 68*: 2227.

Jones, S. F., and Kwanbunbumpen, S. (1970), The effects of nerve stimulation and hemicholinium on synaptic vesicles at the mammalian neuromuscular junction, *J. Physiol. (London) 207*: 31.

Jutisz, M., and Paloma delaLlosa, M. (1970), Requirement of Ca^{++} and Mg^{++} ions for the *in vitro* release of follicle-stimulating hormone from rat pituitary glands and in its subsequent biosynthesis, *Endocrinology 86*: 761.

Kanno, T. (1972), Calcium-dependent amylase release and electrophysiological measurements in cells of the pancreas, *J. Physiol. (London) 226*: 353.

Katz, B. (1958), Microphysiology of the neuromuscular junction, *Bull. Johns Hopkins Hosp. 102*: 275.

Katz. B. (1969), *The Release of Neural Transmitter Substances*, Charles C. Thomas, Springfield, Ill.

Katz, B. (1971), Physiological evidence for quantal transmitter release, *Phil. Trans. Roy. Soc. London B 261*: 381.

Katz, B., and Miledi, R. (1967a), Tetrodotoxin and neuromuscular transmission, *Proc. Roy. Soc. (Ser. B, Biol. Sci.) 167*: 8.

Katz, B., and Miledi, R. (1967b), The timing of calcium action during neuromuscular transmission, *J. Physiol. (London) 189*: 535.

Katz, B., and Miledi, R. (1969), Spontaneous and evoked activity of motor nerve endings in calcium Ringer, *J. Physiol. (London) 203*: 689.

Katz, N. L. (1972), The effects of frog neuromuscular transmission of agents which act upon microtubules and microfilaments, *Europ. J. Pharmacol. 19*: 88.

Katz, R. I., and Kopin, I. J. (1969a), Electrical field-stimulated release of norepinephrine-H^3 from rat atrium: Effects of ions and drugs, *J. Pharmacol. Exptl. Therap. 169*: 229.

Katz, R. I., and Kopin, I. J. (1969b), Release of norepinephrine-^3H and serotonin-^3H evoked from brain slices by electrical-field stimulation—Calcium dependency and the effects of lithium, ouabain and tetrodotoxin, *Biochem. Pharmacol. 18*: 1935.

Kelly, J. S. (1968), The antagonism of Ca^{++} by Na^+ and other monovalent ions at the frog neuromuscular junction, *Quart. J. Exptl. Physiol. 53*: 239.

Kinlough-Rathbone, R. L., Chahil, A., and Mustard, J. F. (1973), Effect of external calcium and magnesium on thrombin-induced changes in calcium and magnesium of pig platelets, *Am. J. Physiol. 224*: 941.

Kirpekar, S. M., and Misu, Y. (1967), Release of noradrenaline by splenic nerve stimulation and its dependence on calcium, *J. Physiol. (London) 188*: 219.

Kirpekar, S. M., Prat, J. C., Puig, M., and Wakade, A. R. (1972), Modification of the evoked release of noradrenaline from the perfused cat spleen by various ions and agents, *J. Physiol. 221*: 601.

Kirshner, N., and Kirshner, A. G. (1971), Chromogranin A, dopamine β-hydroxylase and secretion from the adrenal medulla, *Phil. Trans. Roy. Soc. London B 261*: 279.

Kirshner, N., and Viveros, O. H. (1970), Quantal aspects of the secretion of catecholamines and dopamine-β-hydroxylase from the adrenal medulla, in: *New Aspects of Storage and Release Mechanisms of Catecholamines*, Bayer Symposium, Springer, New York, p. 78.

Kirshner, N., Sage, H. J., and Smith, W. J. (1967), Mechanism of secretion from the adrenal medulla. II. Release of catecholamines and storage vesicle protein in response to chemical stimulation, *Mol. Pharmacol. 3*: 254.

Koefoed-Johnsen, V., and Ussing, H. H. (1953), The contributions of diffusion and flow to the passage of D_2O through living membranes, *Acta Physiol. Scand. 28*: 60.

Koketsu, K., and Nishi, S. (1969), Calcium and action potentials of bullfrog sympathetic ganglion cells, *J. Gen. Physiol. 53*: 608.

Koketsu, K., Kitamura, R., and Tanaka, R. (1964), Binding of calcium ions to cell membrane isolated from bullfrog skeletal muscle, *Am. J. Physiol. 207*: 509.

Kondo, Y., and Ui, W. (1963), A new assay for thyrotropic hormone based on the iodination of thyroglobulin in hog thyroid slices, *Endocrinol. Jap. 10*: 60.

Kopin, I. J., Breese, G. R., Krauss, K. R., and Weise, V. K. (1968), Selective release of newly synthesized norepinephrine from the cat spleen during sympathetic nerve stimulation, *J. Pharmacol. Exptl. Therap. 161*: 271.

Knopp, J., Stolc, V., and Tong, W. (1970), Evidence for the induction of iodide transport in bovine thyroid cells treated with thyroid-stimulating hormone or dibutryryl cyclic adenosine 3′,5′-monophosphate, *J. Biol. Chem. 245*: 4403.

Kraicer, J., and Milligan, J. V. (1971), Effect of colchicine on *in vitro* ACTH release induced by high K^+ and by hypothalamus-stalk–median eminence extract, *Endocrinology 89*: 408.

Kregenow, F. M., and Hoffman, J. F. (1972), Some kinetic and metabolic characteristics of calcium-induced potassium transport in human red cells, *J. Gen. Physiol. 60*: 406.

Kudo, C. F., Rubinstein, D., McKenzie, J. M., and Beck, J. C. (1972), Hormonal release by dispersed pituitary cells, *Can. J. Physiol. Pharmacol. 50*: 860.

Kulka, R. G., and Sternlicht, E. (1968), Enzyme secretion in mouse pancreas mediated by adenosine 3′,5′-cyclic phosphate and inhibited by adenosine 3′-phosphate, *Proc. Natl. Acad. Sci. 61*: 1123.

Kuperman, A. S., Okamoto, M., and Gallin, E. (1967), Nucleotide action on spontaneous electrical activity of calcium deficient nerve, *J. Cell. Physiol. 70*: 257.

Kuriyama, H. (1964), Effect of calcium and magnesium on neuromuscular transmission in the hypogastric nerve–vas deferens preparation of the guinea pig, *J. Physiol. (London) 175*: 211.

Labrie, F., Lemaire, S., and Courte, C. (1971), Adenosine 3′,5′-monophosphate-dependent protein kinase from bovine anterior pituitary gland, *J. Biol. Chem. 246*: 7293.

Lacy, P. E., Howell, S. L., Young, D. A., and Fink, C. J. (1968), New hypothesis of insulin secretion, *Nature 219*: 1177.

Lacy, P. E., Walker, M. M., and Fink, C. J. (1972), Perifusion of isolated rate islets *in vitro*. Participation of the microtubular system in the biphasic release of insulin, *Diabetes 21*: 987.

Lagercrantz, H. (1971), Isolation and characterization of sympathetic nerve trunk vesicles, *Acta Physiol. Scand. Suppl. 366*: 1.

Lambert, A. E., Jeanrenaud, B., Junod, A., and Renold, A. E. (1969a), Organ culture of fetal rat pancreas. II. Insulin release induced by amino and organic acids, by hormonal peptides, by cationic alterations of the medium and by other agents, *Biochim. Biophys. Acta 174*: 540.

Lambert, A. E., Junod, A., Stauffacher, W., Jeanrenaud, B., and Renold, A. E. (1969b), Organ culture of fetal rat pancrease. I. Insulin release induced by caffeine and by sugars and some derivatives, *Biochim. Biophys. Acta 184*: 529.

Landowne, D., and Ritchie, J. M. (1971), On the control of glycogenolysis in mammalian nervous tissue by calcium, *J. Physiol. (London) 212*: 503.

Langer, G. A. (1968), Ion fluxes in cardiac excitation and contraction in their relation to myocardial contractility, *Physiol. Rev. 48*: 708.

Langer, G. A., and Frank, J. S. (1972), Lanthanum in heart cell culture: Effect on calcium exchange correlated with its localization, *J. Cell Biol. 54*: 441.

Lehninger, A. L. (1970), Mitochondria and calcium ion transport, *Biochem. J. 119*: 129.

Levine, R. A., and Wilson, D. E. (1971), The role of cyclic AMP in gastric secretion, *Ann. N.Y. Acad. Sci. 185*: 363.

Lichtenstein, L. M. (1971), The role of cyclic AMP in inhibiting the IgE-mediated release of histamine, *Ann. N.Y. Acad. Sci. 185*: 403.

Liley, A. W. (1956), The effects of presynaptic polarization on the spontaneous activity at the mammalian-neuromuscular junction, *J. Physiol. (London) 134*: 427.

Lipicky, R. J., Hertz, L., and Shanes, A. M. (1963), Ca^{45} transfer and acetylcholine release in the rabbit superior cervical ganglion, *J. Cell. Comp. Physiol. 62*: 233.

Locke, F. S. (1894), Notiz über den Einfluss physiologischer Kochsalzlösung auf die elektrische Erregbarkeit von Muskel und Nerv, *Zentrabl. Physiol. 8*: 166.

Lockhart Ewart, R. B., and Taylor, K. W. (1971), The regulation of growth hormone secretion from the isolated rat anterior pituitary *in vitro, Biochem. J. 124*: 815.

Loeffler, L. J., Lovenberg, W., and Sjoerdsma, A. (1971), Effects of dibutyryl-3′,5′-cyclic adenosine monophosphate, phosphodiesterase inhibitors and prostaglandin E₁ on compound 48/80-induced histamine release from rat peritoneal mast cells *in vitro, Biochem. Pharmacol. 20*: 2287.

Loewi, O. (1921), Über humorale Ubertragbarkeit der Herznervenwirkung, *Pflügers Arch. Ges. Physiol. 189*: 239.

Loewi, O. (1945), Chemical transmission of nerve impulses, *Am. Scientist 33*: 159.

Longenecker, H. E., Hurlbut, W. P., Mauro, A., and Clark, A. W. (1970), Effects of black widow spider venom on the frog neuromuscular junction, *Nature 225*: 701.

Lucke, B., and McCutcheon, M. (1932), The living cell as an osmotic system and its permeability to water, *Physiol. Rev. 12*: 68.

Lundberg, A. (1958), Electrophysiology of salivary glands, *Physiol. Rev. 38*: 21.

Lüscher, E. F., Probst, E., and Bettex-Galland, M. (1972), Thrombostenin: Structure and function, *Ann. N.Y. Acad. Sci. 201*: 122.

Lüttgau, H. C., and Niedergerke, R. (1958), The antagonism between Ca and Na ions on the frog's heart, *J. Physiol. (London) 143*: 486.

MacLeod, R. M., and Fontham, E. H. (1970), Influence of ionic environment on the *in vitro* synthesis and relase of pituitary hormones, *Endocrinology 86*: 863.

MacLeod, R. M., and Lehmeyer, J. E. (1970), Release of pituitary growth hormone by prostaglandins and dibutyryl adenosine cyclic 3′,5′-monophosphate in the absence of protein synthesis, *Proc. Natl. Acad. Sci. 67*: 1172.

Madeira, V. M. C., and Carvalho, A . P. (1972), Interaction of cations and local anesthetics with isolated sarcolemma, *Biochim. Biophys. Acta 266*: 670.

Maizels, M. (1956), Sodium transfer in tortoise erythrocytes, *J. Physiol. (London) 132*: 414.

Malaisse, W. J. (1972), Role of calcium in insulin secretion, *Israel J. Med. Sci. 8*: 244.

Malaisse, W. J., Malaisse-Lagae, F., and Mayhew, D. (1967), A possible role for the adenyl cyclase system in insulin secretion, *J. Clin. Invest. 46*: 1724.

Malaisse, W. J., Malaisse-Lagae, F., and Brisson, G. (1971a), The stimulus–secretion coupling of glucose-induced insulin release. II. Interaction of alkali and alkaline earth cations, *Horm. Met. Res. 3*: 71.

Malaisse, W. J., Malaisse-Lagae, F., Walker, M. O., and Lacy, P. E. (1971b), The stimulus–secretion coupling of glucose-induced insulin release. V. The participation of a microtubular-microfilamentous system, *Diabetes 20*: 257.

Malawista, S. E. (1971), Vinblastine: Colchicine-like effects on human blood leukocytes during phagocytosis, *Blood 37*: 519.

Manery, J. F. (1966), Effects of Ca ions on membranes, *Fed. Proc. 25*: 1804.

Manthey, A. A. (1972), The antagonistic effects of calcium and potassium on the time course of action of carbamycholine at the neuromuscular junction, *J. Membrane Biol. 9*: 319.

Mao, C. C., Shanbour, L. L., Hodgins, D. S., and Jacobson, E. D. (1972), Adenosine 3′,5′-monophosphate (cyclic AMP) and secretion in the canine stomach, *Gastroenterology 63*: 427.

Margolis, R. K., Jaanus, S. D., and Margolis, R. U. (1973), Stimulation by acetylcholine of sulfated mucopolysaccharide release from the perfused cat adrenal gland, *Mol. Pharmacol. 9*: 590.

Margolis, R. U., and Margolis, R. K. (1973), Isolation of chondroitin sulfate and glycopeptides from chromaffin granules of adrenal medulla, *Biochem. Pharmacol. 22*: 2195.

Marquis, N. R., Vigdahl, R. L., and Tavormina, P. A. (1969), Platelet aggregation. I. Regulation by cyclic AMP and prostaglandin E_1, *Biochem. Biophys. Res. Commun. 36*: 965.

Martinez, J. R., and Petersen, O. H. (1972), The importance of extracellular calcium for acetylcholine-evoked salivery secretion, *Experientia 28*: 167.

Matthews, E. K. (1967), Membrane potential measurement in cells of the adrenal gland, *J. Physiol. (London) 189*: 139.

Matthews, E. K., and Petersen, O. H. (1973), Pancreatic acinar cells: Ionic dependence of the membrane potential and acetylcholine-induced depolarization, *J. Physiol. (London) 231*: 283.

Matthews, E. K., and Saffran, M. (1967), Steroid production and membrane potential measurement in cells of the adrenal cortex, *J. Physiol. (London) 189*: 149.

Matthews, E. K., and Saffran, M. (1968), Effect of ACTH on the electrical properties of adrenocortical cells, *Nature 219*: 1369.

Matthews, E. K., Evans, R. J., and Dean, P. M. (1972), The ionogenic nature of the secretory-granule membrane, *Biochem. J. 130*: 825.

Mazia, D. (1940), The binding of ions by the cell surface, *Cold Spring Harbor Symp. 8*: 195.

Meech, R. W. (1972), Intracellular calcium injection causes increased potassium conductance in *Aplysia* nerve cells, *Comp. Biochem. Physiol. 42*: 493.

Meiri, U., and Rahamimoff, R. (1972), Neuromuscular transmission: Inhibition by manganese ions, *Science 176*: 308.

Meis de, L., Rubin-Altschul, B., and Machado, R. D. (1970), Comparative data of Ca^{2+} transport in brain and skeletal muscle microsomes, *J. Biol. Chem. 245*: 1883.

Mela, L. (1969), Inhibition and activation of calcium transport in mitochondria: Effect of lanthanides and local anesthetic drugs, *Biochemistry 8*: 2481.

Miledi, R. (1071), Lanthanum ions abolish the "calcium response" of nerve terminal, *Nature 229*: 410.

Miledi, R., and Slater, C. R. (1966), The action of calcium on neuronal synapses in the squid, *J. Physiol. (London) 184*: 473

Milligan, J. V., and Kraicer, J. (1970), Adenohypophysial transmembrane potentials: Polarity reversal by elevated external potassium ion concentration, *Science 167*: 182.

Milligan, J. V., and Kraicer, J. (1972), Purified growth hormone releasing factor increases ^{45}Ca uptake into pituitary cells, *Can. J. Physiol. Pharmacol. 50*: 613.

Milner, R. D. G. (1970), The stimulation of insulin release by essential amino acids from rabbit pancreas *in vitro*, *J. Endocrinol. 47*: 347.

Milner, R. D. G., and Hales, C. N. The interaction of various inhibitors and stimuli of insulin release studied with rabbit pancreas *in vitro*, *Biochem. J. 113*: 473.

Mines, G. R. (1911), On the replacement of calcium in certain neuromuscular mechanisms by allied substances, *J. Physiol. (London) 42*: 251.

Mongar, J. L., and Schild, H. O. (1958), The effect of calcium and pH on the anaphylactic reaction, *J. Physiol. (London) 140*: 72.

Montague, W., and Cook, J. R. (1971), The role of adenosine 3′,5′-cyclic monophosphate in the regulation of insulin release by isolated rat islets of Langerhans, *Biochem. J. 122*: 115.

Montague, W., and Howell, S. L. (1973), The mode of action of adenosine 3′,5′-cyclic monophosphate in mammalian islets of Langerhans, *Biochem. J. 134*: 321.

Morisset, J. A., and Webster, P. D. (1971), *In vitro* and *in vivo* effects of pancreozymin, urecholine and cyclic AMP on rat pancreas, *Am. J. Physiol. 220*: 202.

Mürer, E. H. (1971), Compounds known to affect the cyclic adenosine monophosphate level in blood platelets: Effect on thrombin-induced clot retraction and platelet release, *Biochim. Biophys. Acta 237*: 310.

Mürer, E. H., and Holme, R. (1970), A study of the release of calcium from human blood platelets and its inhibition by metabolic inhibitors, N-ethylmaleimide and aspirin, *Biochim. Biophys. Acta 222*: 197.

Musick, J., and Hubbard, J. I. (1972), Release of protein from mouse motor nerve terminals, *Nature 237*: 279.

Mustard, J. F., and Packham, M. A. (1970), Factors influencing platelet function: Adhesion, release and aggregation, *Pharmacol. Rev. 22*: 97.

Nadler, N. J. (1971), Anatomy and histochemistry of the thyroid, in: *The Thyroid* (S. C. Werner and S. H. Ingbar, eds.), Harper and Row, New York, p. 9.

Nagasawa, H., and Yanai, R. (1972), Promotion of pituitary prolactin release in rats by dibutyryl adenosine 3′,5′-monophosphate, *J. Endocrinol. 55*: 215.

Nash, C. W., Tu, T., and Martin, M. J. (1972), The influence of inorganic ions on the uptake and retention of tritiated noradrenaline by isolated perfused rat hearts, *Can. J. Physiol. Pharmacol. 50*: 645.

Nayler, W. G. (1966), Influx and efflux of calcium in the physiology of muscle contraction, *Clin. Orthop. Rel. Res. 46*: 157.

Nickel, E., and Potter, L. T. (1971), Synaptic vesicles in freeze-etched electric tissue of *Torpedo*, *Phil. Trans. Roy. Soc. London B 261*: 383.

Niedergerke, R. (1963), Movements of Ca in frog heart ventricles at rest and during contractures, *J. Physiol. (London) 167*: 515.

Niedergerke, R., and Orkland, R. K. (1966), The dual effect of calcium on the actual potential of the frog's heart, *J. Physiol. (London) 184*: 291.

Nielsen, S. P., and Petersen, O. H. (1972), Transport of calcium in the perfused submandibular gland of the cat, *J. Physiol. (London) 223*: 685.

Ohnishi, T., and Ebashi, S. (1963), Spectrophotometrical measurement of instantaneous calcium binding of the relaxing factor of muscle, *J. Biochem. (Tokyo) 54*: 506.

Olmsted, J. B., and Borisy, G. G. (1973), Microtubules, *Ann. Rev. Biochem. 42*: 507.

Orci, L., Gabbay, K. H., and Malaisse, W. J. (1971), Pancreatic beta-cell web: Its possible role in insulin secretion, *Science 175*: 1128.

Orr, T. S. C., Hall, D. E., and Allison, A. C. (1972), Role of contractile microfilaments in the release of histamine from mast cells, *Nature 236*: 350.

Otsuka, M., Iversen, L. L., Hall, Z. W., and Kravitz, E. A. (1966), Release of gamma-aminobutyric acid from inhibitory nerves of lobster, *Proc. Natl. Acad. Sci. 56*: 1110.

Palade, G. E. (1959), Functional changes in the structure of cell components, in: *Subcellular Particles* (T. Hayashi, ed.), Ronald Press, New York.

Palmer, R. F., and Posey, V. A. (1970), Calcium and adenosine triphosphate binding to renal membranes, *J. Gen. Physiol. 55*: 89.

Papahadjopoulos, D. (1972), Studies on the mechanism of action of local anesthetics with phospholipid model membranes, *Biochim. Biophys. Acta 265*: 169.

Pappano, A. J., and Volle, R. L. (1966), Observations on the role of calcium ions in ganglionic responses to acetylcholine, *J. Pharmacol. Exptl. Therap. 152*: 171.

Parsons, J. A. (1970), Effects of cations on prolactin and growth hormone secretion by rat adenohypophyses *in vitro, J. Physiol. (London) 210*: 973.

Pastan, I., and Macchia, V. (1967), Mechanism of thyroid-stimulating hormone action: Studies with dibutyryl 3′,5′-adenosine monophosphate and lecithinase C, *J. Biol. Chem. 242*: 5757.

Paton, W. D. M., and Rothschild, A. M. (1965), The effect of varying calcium concentration on the kinetic constants of hyoscine and mepyramine antagonism, *Brit. J. Pharmacol. 24*: 432.

Patriarca, P. and Carafoli, E. (1968), A study of the intracellular transport of calcium in rat heart, *J. Cell. Physiol. 72*: 29.

Patt, H. M., and Luckhardt, A. B. (1942), Relationship of a low blood calcium to parathyroid secretion, *Endocrinology 31*: 384.

Peach, M. J. (1972), Stimulation of release of adrenal catecholamine by adenosine 3′,5′-cyclic monophosphate and theophylline in the absence of extracellular Ca^{++}, *Proc. Natl. Acad. Sci. 69*: 834.

Pelletier, G., Lemay, A., Beraud, G., and Labrie, F. (1972), Ultrastructural changes accompanying the stimulatory effect of N^6-monobutyryl adenosine 3′,5′-monophosphate on the release of growth hormone (GH), prolactin

(PRL) and adrenocorticotropic hormone (ACTH) in rat anterior pituitary gland *in vitro, Endocrinology 91*: 1355.

Peron, F. G., and McCarthy, J. L. (1968), Corticosteroidogenesis in the rat adrenal gland, in: *Functions of the Adrenal Cortex*, Vol. 1 (K. W. McKerns, ed.), Appleton-Century-Crofts, New York, p. 261.

Petersen, O. H. (1970), The importance of extracellular sodium and potassium for acetylcholine-evoked salivary secretion, *Experientia 26*: 1103.

Petersen, O. H. (1971), The ionic transports involved in the acetylcholine-induced change in membrane potential in acinar cells from salivary glands and their importance in the salivary secretion process, in: *Electrophysiology of Epithelial Cells* (G. Giebisch, ed.), Schattaver Verlag, New York, p. 207.

Petersen, O. H. (1972), Acetylcholine-induced ion transports involved in the formation of saliva, *Acta Physiol. Scand. Suppl. 381*.

Petersen, O. H., and Matthews, E. K. (1972), The effect of pancreozymin and acetylcholine on the membrane potential of the pancreatic acinar cells, *Experientia 28*: 1037.

Petersen, O. H., and Poulsen, J. H. (1967), The effects of varying the extracellular potassium concentration on the secretory rate and on the resting and secretory potentials in the perfused cat submandibular gland, *Acta Physiol. Scand. 70*: 293.

Petersen, O. H., Poulsen, J. H., and Thorn, N. A. (1967), Secretory potentials, secretory rate, and water permeability of the duct system in the cat submandibular gland during perfusion with calcium-free Locke's solution, *Acta Physiol. Scand. 71*: 203.

Pickup, J. C., Johnston, C. I., Nakamura, S., Uttenthal, L. O., and Hope, D. B. (1973), Subcellular organization of neurophysins, oxytocin, [8-lysine]-vasopressin and adenosine triphosphatase in porcine pituitary lobes, *Biochem. J. 132*: 361.

Poisner, A. M. (1970), Release of transmitters from storage: A contractile model, *Advan. Biochem. Psychopharmacol. 2*: 95.

Poisner, A. M. (1973), Stimulus–secretion coupling in the adrenal medulla and posterior pituitary gland, in: *Frontiers in Neuroendocrinology* (W. F. Ganong and L. Martini, eds.), Oxford University Press, New York, p. 33.

Poisner, A. M., and Bernstein, J. (1971), A possible role of microtubules in catecholamines release from the adrenal medulla: Effect of colchicine, vinca alkaloids and deuterium oxide, *J. Pharmacol. Exptl. Therap. 177*: 102.

Poisner, A. M., and Douglas, W. W. (1968), A possible mechanism of release of posterior pituitary hormones involving adenosine triphosphate and an adenosine triphosphatase in the neurosecretory granules, *Mol. Pharmacol. 4*: 531.

Poisner, A. M., and Trifaro, J. M. (1967), The role of ATP and ATPase in the release of catecholamines from the adrenal medulla. I. ATP-evoked release of catecholamines, ATP, and protein from isolated chromaffin granules, *Mol. Pharmacol. 3*: 561.

Poste, G., and Allison, A. C. (1971), Membrane fusion reaction: A theory, *J. Theoret. Biol. 32*: 165.

Prince, W. T., Berridge, M. J., and Ramussen, H. (1972), Role of calcium and adenosine-3',5'-cyclic monophosphate in controlling fly salivary gland secretion, *Proc. Natl. Acad. Sci.* 69: 553.

Quastel, D. M. J., Hackett, J. T., and Cooke, J. D. (1971), Calcium: Is it required for transmitter secretion? *Science 172*: 1034.

Rahamimoff, R. (1970), Role of calcium ions in neuromuscular transmission, in: *Calcium and Cellular Function* (A. W. Cuthbert, ed.), Macmillan, London, p. 131.

Rall, T. W., Sutherland, E. W., and Berthet, J. (1957), The relationship of epinephrine and glucagon to liver phosphosphorylase. IV. Effect of epinephrine and glucagon on the reactivation of phosphorylase in liver homogenates, *J. Biol. Chem.* 224: 463.

Ramwell, P. W., and Rabinowitz, I. (1972), Interaction of prostaglandins and cyclic AMP, in: *Effect of Drugs on Cellular Control Mechanisms* (B. R. Rabin and R. B. Freedman, eds.), University Park Press, Baltimore, p. 207.

Ramwell, P. W., and Shaw, J. E. (1970), Biological significance of the prostaglandins, *Rec. Prog. Horm. Res. 26*: 139.

Randle, P. J., and Hales, C. N. (1972), Insulin release mechanisms, in: *Handbook of Physiology*, Sect. 7: *Endocrinology*, Vol. I: *Endocrine Pancreas* (D. F. Steiner and N. Freinkel,eds.), American Physiological Society, Washington, D.C., p. 219.

Rasmussen, H. (1970), Cell communication, calcium ion, and cyclic adenosine monophosphate, *Science 170*: 404.

Rasmussen, H., and Nagata, N. (1970), Hormones, cell calcium and cyclic AMP, in: *Calcium and Cellular Function* (A. W. Cuthbert, ed.), Macmillan, London, p. 198.

Rasmussen, H., and Tenenhouse, A. (1968), Cyclic adenosine monophosphate, Ca^{++}, and membranes, *Proc. Natl. Acad. Sci. 59*: 1364.

Redburn, D. A., Poisner, A. M., and Samson, F. E. (1972), Comparison of microtubule protein (tubulin) from adrenal medulla and brain, *Brain Res. 44*: 615.

Reuter, H. (1970), Kinetic aspects of calcium current in ventricular myocardial fibres, in: *Calcium and Cellular Function* (A. W. Cuthbert, ed.), Macmillan, London, p. 261.

Reuter, H., and Seitz, N. (1968), The dependence of calcium efflux from cardiac muscle on temperature and external ion composition, *J. Physiol. (London) 195*: 451.

Ridderstap, A. S., and Bonting, S. L. (1969), Cyclic AMP and enzyme secretion by the isolated rabbit pancreas, *Pflügers Arch. Ges. Physiol. 313*: 62.

Ringer, S. (1883), A further contribution regarding the influence of the different constituents of the blood on the contraction of the heart, *J. Physiol. (London) 4*: 29.

Ringer, S. (1890), Concerning experiments to test the influence of lime, sodium and potassium salts on the development of ova and growth of tadpoles, *J. Physiol. (London) 11*: 79.

Ritchie, J. M. (1965), The action of acetylcholine and related drugs on mammalian non-myelinated nerve fibers, in: *Pharmacology of Cholinergic and Adrenergic Transmission* (G. B. Koelle, W. W. Douglas, and A. Carlsson, eds.), Macmillan, New York, p. 55.

Robinson, J. D., and Lust, W. D. (1968), Adenosine triphosphate-dependent calcium accumulation by brain microsomes, *Arch. Biochem. Biophys. 125*: 286.

Robison, G. A., Butcher, R. W., and Sutherland, E. W. (1971), *Cyclic AMP*, Academic Press, New York.

Röhlich, P., Anderson, P., and Uvnäs, B. (1971), Electron microscope observations on compound 48/80-induced degranulation in rat mast cells, *J. Cell Biol. 51*: 465.

Rojas, E., Taylor, R. E., Atwater, I., and Bezanilla, F. (1969), Analysis of the effects of calcium or magnesium on voltage-clamp currents in perfused squid axons bathed in solutions of high potassium, *J. Gen. Physiol. 54*: 532.

Rossignol, B., Herman, G., and Keryer, G. (1972), Inhibition by colchicine of carbamylcholine induced glycoprotein secretion by the submaxillary gland: A possible mechanism of cholinergic induced protein secretion, *FEBS Letters 21*: 189.

Rubin, M. (1963), The biological implications of alkaline earth chelation, in: *The Transfer of Calcium and Strontium Across Biological Membranes* (R. H. Wasserman, ed.), Academic Press, New York, p. 25.

Rubin, R. P. (1969), The metabolic requirements for catecholamine release from the adrenal medulla, *J. Physiol. (London) 202*: 197.

Rubin, R. P. (1970), The role of calcium in the release of neurotransmitter substances and hormones, *Pharmacol. Rev. 22*: 389.

Rubin, R. P., and Miele, E. (1968), A study of the differential secretion of epinephrine and norepinephrine from the perfused cat adrenal gland, *J. Pharmacol. Exptl. Therap. 164*: 115.

Rubin, R. P., Feinstein, M. B., Jaanus, S. D., and Paimre, M. (1967), Inhibition of catecholamine secretion and calcium exchange in perfused cat adrenal glands by tetracaine and magnesium, *J. Pharmacol. Exptl. Therap. 155*: 463.

Rubin, R. P., Jaanus, S. D., and Carchman, R. A. (1972), Role of calcium and adenosine cyclic 3′,5′-phosphate in action of adrenocorticotropin, *Nature 240*: 150.

Salzman, E. W., Kensler, P. C., and Levine, L. (1972), Cyclic 3′,5′-adenosine monophosphate in human blood platelets. IV. Regulatory role of cyclic AMP in platelet function, *Ann. N.Y. Acad. Sci. 201*: 61.

Samli, M. H., and Geschwind, I. I. (1968), Some effects of energy-transfer inhibitors and of Ca^{++}-free or K^+-enhanced media on the release of luteinizing hormone (LH) from the rat pituitary gland *in vitro*, *Endocrinology 82*: 225.

Saruta, T., and Kaplan, N. M. (1972), Adrenocortical steroidogenesis: The effects of prostaglandins, *J. Clin. Invest. 51*: 2246.

Sato, S., Szabo, M., Kowalski, K., and Burke, G. (1972), Role of prostaglandin in thyrotropin action on thyroid, *Endocrinology 90*: 343.

Schally, A. V., Arimura, A., and Kastin, A. J. (1973), Hypothalamic regulatory hormones, *Science 179*: 341.

Schatzmann, H. J. (1970), Transmembrane calcium movements in resealed human red cells, in: *Calcium and Cellular Function* (A. W. Cuthbert, ed.), Macmillan, London, p. 85.

Schell-Frederick, E., and Dumont, J. E. (1970), Mechanism of action of thyrotropin, in: *Biochemical Actions of Hormones,* Vol. I (G. Litwack, ed.), Academic Press, New York, p. 415.

Schmitt, F. O. (1968), Fibrous proteins—Neuronal organelles, *Proc. Natl. Acad. Sci. 60*: 1092.

Schneider, F. (1972), Amphetamine-induced exocytosis of catecholamines from the cow adrenal medulla, *J. Pharmacol. Exptl. Therap. 183*: 80.

Schneyer, L. H. (1967), Exchange of potassium in rat submaxillary gland, in: *Secretory Mechanisms of Salivary Glands* (L. H. Schneyer and C. A. Schneyer, eds.), Academic Press, New York, p. 32.

Schneyer, L. H., Young, J. A., and Schneyer, C. (1972), Salivary secretion of electrolytes, *Physiol. Rev. 52*: 720.

Schramm, M. (1968), Amylase secretion in rat parotid slices by apparent activation of endogenous catecholamine, *Biochim. Biophys. Acta 165*: 546.

Selinger, Z., and Naim, E. (1970), The effect of calcium on amylase secretion by rat parotid slices, *Biochim. Biophys. Acta 203*: 335.

Selinger, Z., Naim, E., and Lasser, M. (1970), ATP-dependent calcium uptake by microsomal preparations from rat parotid and submaxillary glands, *Biochim. Biophys. Acta 203*: 326.

Shanes, A. M. (1958), Electrochemical aspects in excitable cells, *Pharmacol. Rev. 10*: 59.

Shanes, A. M. (1961), Calcium influx in frog rectus abdominis muscle at rest and during potassium contracture, *J. Cell. Comp. Physiol. 57*: 193.

Shanes, A. M., and Bianchi, C. P. (1959), The distribution and kinetics of release of radiocalcium in tendon and skeletal muscle, *J. Gen. Physiol. 42*: 1123.

Shaw, J. E., and Ramwell, P. W. (1968), Inhibition of gastric secretion in rats by prostaglandin E_1 in: *Prostaglandin Symposium of the Worcester Foundation for Experimental Biology* (P. W. Ramwell and J. E. Shaw, eds.), Interscience, New York, p. 55.

Sherwood, L. M., Mayer, G. P., Ramberg, C. F., Kronfeld, D. S., Aurbach, G. D., and Potts, J. T. (1968), Regulation of parathyroid hormone secretion: Proportional control by calcium, lack of effect of phosphate, *Endocrinology 83*: 1043.

Sherwood, L. M., Herrman, I., and Bassett, C. A. (1970), Parathyroid hormone secretion *in vitro*: Regulation by calcium and magnesium ions, *Nature 225*: 1056.

Slorach, S. A., and Uvnäs, B. (1969), Dissociation of histamine release and $^{22}Na^+$ uptake in rat mast cells exposed to compound 48/80 *in vitro*, *Acta Physiol. Scand. 76*: 201.

Smallwood, R. A. (1967), Effects of intravenous calcium administration on gastric secretion of acid and pepsin in man, *Gut 8*: 592.

Smith, A. D. (1971), Secretion of proteins (chromogranin A and dopamine β-hydroxylase) from a sympathetic neuron, *Phil. Trans. Roy. Soc. London B 261*: 363.

Smith, A. D. (1972), Storage and secretion of hormones, in: *The Scientific Basis of Medicine: Annual Reviews*, The Athlone Press, London, p. 74.

Smith, A. D., and Winkler, H. (1972), Fundamental mechanisms in the release of catecholamines, in: *Handbook of Experimental Pharmacology*, Vol. XXXIII (H. Blaschko and E. Muscholl, eds.) Springer-Verlag, Berlin, p. 538.

Smith, V., Smith, D. S., Winkler, H., and Ryan, J. W. (1973), Exocytosis in the adrenal medulla demonstrated by freeze-etching, *Science 179*: 79.

Sneddon, J. M. (1972), Divalent cations and the blood platelet release reaction, *Nature 236*: 103.

Solomon, A. M. (1962), Ion transport in single cell populations, Proceedings of a Symposium Presented at the International Biophysics Congress, *Biophys. J. 2*: 79.

Somlyo, A. P., and Somlyo, A. V. (1968), Vascular smooth muscle, *Pharmacol. Rev. 20*: 197.

Sorimachi, M., Oesch, F., and Thoenen, H. (1973), Effects of colchicine and cytochalasin on the release of ^3H-norepinephrine from guinea-pig atria evoked by high potassium, nicotine and tyramine, *Naunyn-Schmiedebergs Arch. Pharmakol. 276*: 1.

Stahl, W. L., and Swanson, P. D. (1972), Calcium movements in brain slices in low sodium or calcium media, *J. Neurochem. 19*: 2395.

Statland, B. E., Heagan, B. M., and White, J. G. (1969), Uptake of calcium by platelet relaxing factor, Nature 223: 521.

Steiner, A. L., Peake, G. T., Utiger, R. D., Karl, I. E., and Kipnis, D. M. (1970), Hypothalamic stimulation of growth hormone and thyrotropin release *in vitro* and pituitary $3',5'$-adenosine cyclic monophosphate, *Endocrinology 86*: 1354.

Strandberg, K. (1971), Ca^{++} dependence of histamine release and formation of slow reacting substance in the cat paw, *Acta Physiol. Scand. 82*: 500.

Sugiyama, K. (1971), Calcium-dependent histamine release with degranulation from isolated rat mast cells by adenosine $5'$-triphosphate, *Jap. J. Pharmacol. 21*: 209.

Sulakhe, P. V., and Dhalla, N. S. (1970), Excitation–contraction coupling in heart. III. Evidence against the involvement of adenosine cyclic $3',5'$-monophosphate in calcium transport by sarcotubular vesicles of canine myocardium, *Mol. Pharmacol. 6*: 659.

Sundberg, D. K., Krulich, L., Fawcett, C. P., Illner, P., and McCann, S. M. (1973), The effect of colchicine on the release of rat anterior pituitary hormones *in vitro, Proc. Soc. Exptl. Biol. 142*: 1097.

Takata, M., Pickard, W. F., Lettvin, J. Y., and Moore, S. W. (1966), Ionic conductance changes in lobster axon membrane when lanthanum is substituted for calcium, *J. Gen. Physiol. 50*: 461.

Takeuchi, N. (1963), Effects of calcium on the conductance change of the end-plate membrane during the action of transmitter, *J. Physiol. (London) 167*: 141.

Tasaki, K., Sugiyama, K., Komoto, S., and Yamasaki, H. (1970), Dissociation of degranulation and depolarization of the rat mesentery mast cell exposed to compound 48/80 and ATP, *Proc. Jap. Acad. 46*: 826.

Temple, R., Williams, J. A., Wilber, J. F., and Wolff, J. (1972), Colchicine and hormone secretion, *Biochem. Biophys. Res. Commun. 46*: 1454.

Thiers, R. E., Reynolds, E. S., and Vallee, B. L. (1960), The effect of carbon tetrachloride poisoning on subcellular metal distribution in rat liver, *J. Biol. Chem. 235*: 2130.

Thoenen, H., Huerlimann, A., and Haefely, W. (1969), Cation dependence of the noradrenaline-releasing action of tyramine, *Europ. J. Pharmacol. 6*: 29.

Thon, I. L., and Uvnäs, B. (1967), Degranulation and histamine release, two consecutive steps in the response of rat mast cells to compound 48/80, *Acta Physiol. Scand. 71*: 303.

Tidball, M. E., and Scherer, R. W. (1972), Relationship of calcium and magnesium to platelet histamine release, *Am. J. Physiol. 222*: 1303.

Tidball, M. E., Scherer, R. W., and Levy, A. G. (1971), Platelet sodium, potassium and histamine translocation during histamine release, *Am. J. Physiol. 221*: 1064.

Tobias, J. M. (1964), A chemically specified molecular mechanism underlying excitation in nerve: A hypothesis, *Nature 203*: 13.

Trautwein, W., and Dudel, J. (1958), Zum Mechanismus der Membranwirkung des Acetylcholin und der Herzmuskelfaser, *Pflugers Arch. Ges. Physiol. 226*: 324.

Trifaro, J. M., Collier, B., Lastowecka, A., and Stern, D. (1972), Inhibition by colchicine and by vinblastine of acetylcholine-induced catecholamine release from the adrenal gland: An anticholinergic action, not an effect upon microtubules, *Mol. Pharmacol. 8*: 264.

Trudeau, W. L., and McGuigan, J. E. (1969), Effects of calcium on serum gastrin levels in the Zollinger-Ellison syndrome, *New Engl. J. Med. 281*: 862.

Tuttle, R. R., and Moran, N. C. (1969), The effect of calcium depletion on the combination of agonists and competitive antagonists with α-adrenergic and histaminergic receptors of rabbit aorta, *J. Pharmacol. Exptl. Therap. 169*: 255.

Usherwood, P. N. R., Machili, P., and Leaf, G. (1968), L-Glutamate at insect excitatory nerve–muscle synapses, *Nature 219*: 1169.

Uttenthal, L. O., Livett, B. G., and Hope, D. B. (1971), Release of neurophysin together with vasopressin by a Ca^{+2}-dependent mechanism, *Phil. Trans. Roy. Soc. London B 261*: 379.

Uvnäs, B. (1964), Release processes in mast cells and their activation by injury, *Ann. N.Y. Acad. Sci. 116*: 880.

Uvnäs, B., Aborg, C. H., and Bergendorf, A. (1970), Storage of histamine in mast cells: Evidence for an ionic binding of histamine to protein carboxyls in the granule heparin–protein complex, *Acta Physiol. Scand. 78*: Suppl. 336.

Wakabayashi, K., Kamberi, I. A., and McCann, S. M. (1969), *In vitro* response of the rat pituitary to gonadotrophin-releasing factors and to ions, *Endocrinology 85*: 1046.

Wallach, D., and Schramm, M. (1071), Calcium and the exportable protein in rat parotid gland, *Europ. J. Biochem. 21*: 433.

Walsh, D. A., Perkins, J. P., and Krebs, E. W. (1968), An adenosine 3',5'-monophosphate-dependent protein kinase from rabbit skeletal muscle, *J. Biol. Chem. 243*: 3763.

Watanabe, A., and Tasaki, I. (1971), The biionic action potential and indispensability of divalent cations in the external medium for nerve excitation, in: *Cellular Mechanisms for Calcium Transfer and Homeostasis* (G. Nichols and R. H. Wasserman, eds.), Academic Press, New York, p. 77.

Way, L., and Durbin, R. P. (1969), Inhibition of gastric acid secretion *in vitro* by prostaglandin E_1, *Nature 221*: 874.

Weber, A., Herz, R., and Reiss, I. (1967), Studies of the kinetics of calcium transport by isolated fragmented sarcoplasmic reticulum, *Biochem. Z. 345*: 329.

Weisenberg, R. C., Borisy, G. G., and Taylor, E. W. (1968), The colchicine-binding protein of mammalian brain and its relation to microtubules, *Biochemistry 7*: 4466.

Weiss, G. B., and Bianchi, C. P. (1965), The effect of potassium concentration on Ca^{45} uptake in frog sartorius muscle, *J. Cell. Comp. Physiol. 65*: 385.

Weiss, G. B., and Goodman, F. R. (1969), Effects of lanthanum on contraction calcium distribution and Ca^{45} movements in intestinal smooth muscle, *J. Pharmacol. Exptl. Therap. 169*: 46.

Wilbrandt, W., and Koller, H. (1948), Die Calciumwirkung am Froscherzen als Funktion des Ionengleichgewichts zwischen Zellmembran und Umgebung, *Helv. Physiol. Pharmacol. Acta 6*: 208.

Williams, G. A., Hargis, G. K., Bowser, E. N., Hendersen, W. J., and Martinez, N. J. (1973), Evidence for a role of adenosine 3',5'-monophosphate in parathyroid hormone release, *Endocrinology 92*: 687.

Williams, J. A. (1966), Effects of external K^+ concentration on transmembrane potentials of rabbit thyroid cells, *Am. J. Physiol. 211*: 1171.

Williams, J. A. (1970), Effects of TSH on thyroid membrane properties, *Endocrinology 86*: 1154.

Williams, J. A. (1972a), Effects of Na^+ and K^+ on secretion *in vitro* by mouse thyroid glands, *Endocrinology 90*: 1452.

Williams, J. A. (1972b), Effects of Ca^{++} and Mg^{++} on secretion *in vitro* by mouse thyroid glands, *Endocrinology 90*: 1459.

Williams, J. A., and Wolff, J. (1972), Colchicine-binding protein and the secretion of thyroid hormone, *J. Cell Biol. 54*: 157.

Williams, T. F., Exton, J. H., Friedmann, N., and Park, C. R. (1971), Effects of insulin and adenosine 3',5'-monophosphate on K$^+$ flux and glucose output in perfused rat liver, *Am. J. Physiol. 221*: 1645.

Winkler, H. (1971), The membrane of the chromaffin granule, *Phil. Trans. Roy. Soc. London B 261*: 293.

Winkler, H., Schöpf, J. A. L., Hörtnagl, H., and Hörtnagl, H. (1972), Bovine adrenal medulla: Subcellular distribution of newly synthesized catecholamines, nucleotides and chromogranins, *Naunyn-Schmiedebergs Arch. Pharmakol. 273*: 43.

Woodbury, D. M., and Woodbury, J. W. (1963), Correlation of microelectrode potential recordings with histology of rat and guinea pig thyroid glands, *J. Physiol. (London) 169*: 553.

Woodin, A. M. (1968), The basis of leucocidin action, in: *The Biological Basis of Medicine*, Vol. 2 (E. E. Bitar, ed.), Academic Press, New York, p. 373.

Woodin, A. M., and Wieneke, A. A. (1963), The accumulation of calcium by the polymorphonuclear leucocyte treated with staphylococcal leucocidin and its significance in the extrusion of protein, *Biochem. J. 87*: 487.

Woodin, A. M., and Wieneke, A. A. (1964), The participation of calcium adenosine trophosphate and adenosine triphosphatase in the extrusion of the granular proteins from the polymorphonuclear leucocyte, *Biochem. J. 90*: 498.

Woodin, A. M., and Wieneke, A. A. (1968), Role of leucocidin and triphosphoinositide in the control of potassium permeability, *Nature 220*: 283.

Woodin, A. M., and Wieneke, A. A. (1970), Site of protein secretion and calcium accumulation in the polymorphonuclear leucocyte treated with leucocidin, in: *Calcium and Cellular Function* (A. W. Cuthbert, ed.), Macmillan, London, p. 183.

Woodin, A. M., French, J. E., and Marchesi, V. T. (1963), Morphological changes associated with the extrusion of protein induced in the polymorphonuclear leucocyte by staphylococcal leucocidin, *Biochem. J. 87*: 567.

Wooten, G. F., Thoa, N. B., Kopin, I. J., and Axelrod, J. (1973), Enhanced release of dopamine β-hydroxylase and norepinephrine from sympathetic nerves by dibutyryl cyclic adenosine 3',5'-monophosphate and theophylline, *Mol. Pharmacol. 9*: 178.

Wuerker, R. B., and Kirkpatrick, J. B. (1972), Neuronal microtubules, neurofilaments and microfilaments, *Internat. Rev. Cytol. 33*: 45.

Yoshida, H., Kadota, K., and Fujisawa, H. (1966), Adenosine triphosphate dependent calcium binding of microsomes and nerve endings, *Nature 212*: 291.

Ziance, R. J., Azzaro, A. J., and Rutledge, C. O. (1972), Characteristics of amphetamine-induced release of norepinephrine from rat cerebral cortex *in vitro, J. Pharmacol. Exptl. Therap. 182*: 284.

Zigmond, S. H., and Hirsch, J. G. (1972), Cytochalasin B: Inhibition of D-2-deoxyglucose transport into leukocytes and fibroblasts, *Science 176*: 1432.

Zor, V., Lowe, I. P., Bloom, G., and Field, J. B. (1968), The role of calcium (Ca^{++}) in TSH and dibutyryl 3',5'-cyclic AMP stimulation of thyroid glucose oxidation and phospholipid synthesis, *Biochem. Biophys. Res. Commun. 33*: 649.

Zor, V., Kanedo, T., Schneider, H. P. G., McCann, S. M., and Field, J. B. (1970), Further studies of stimulation of anterior pituitary cyclic adenosine 3',5'-monophosphate formation by hypothalamic extract and prostaglandins, *J. Biol. Chem. 245*: 2883.

Index

Acetylcholine
  induced amylase secretion 72-73
  induced salivary secretion 33, 66-72,
  permeability change produced by 7-9,
    26-32, 35
  release 25-26
    from autonomic fibers 38, 44-51, 74
    from neuromuscular junction 36-40,
      42, 44-51
Actin 66, 117, 122-124
Actomyosin 122-124
  in brain 122
  in muscle 66
  in platelets 66
Adenosine cyclic monophosphate (see
    cyclic AMP)
Adenosine triphosphatase (ATPase)
  calcium-activated 16, 17, 66, 115
  in cytoplasmic motility 122-123
  in erythrocytes 16-17
  in platelets 66
  in sarcoplasmic reticulum 16
  in secretory granules 102, 114-115
  ouabain inhibition of 41, 95
  sodium-activated 12, 41, 95
Adenosine triphosphate (ATP)
  discharge during secretion of
    catecholamines 102, 103
    histamine 58-62
    5-hydroxytryptamine 62-64, 66

Adenosine triphosphate (ATP) *(cont'd)*
  induced release from isolated granules
    114-115
  in erythrocytes 16-17
  in secretory granules 62, 63, 102
  interaction with calcium 19, 20, 76,
    114, 122-124
Adenylate cyclase 125, 137, 145
  and calcium 148-149
Adhesion, cell 2
Adrenal cortex 87-89, 147-149
  calcium concentration 51
  effects of ACTH on 87-89
  effects of cyclic AMP on 128, 133, 134,
    137, 138, 139, 141, 142
  steroidogenesis
    effects of cations on 87-89, 147-149
Adrenal medulla 26-32, 44-49, 74, 80,
    85, 101-108. 114, 119, 120
  and cyclic AMP 131, 134, 135, 136,
    141
  calcium concentration 5
Adrenergic synapses 54-58, 105-108,
    109, 120
  role of cyclic AMP 135, 136
Adrenocorticotropin (ACTH)
  actions mediated by calcium 147-149
  actions mediated by cyclic AMP 127
  on cyclic AMP levels 138, 147-149
  release of 92-96